Information and IT for Primary Care

EVERYTHING YOU NEED TO KNOW BUT ARE AFRAID TO ASK

Alan Gillies

Professor in Information Management
University of Central Lancashire

Radcliffe Medical Press

© 2000 Alan Gillies

Radcliffe Medical Press Ltd
18 Marcham Road, Abingdon, Oxon OX14 1AA

British Library Cataloguing in Publication Data

A catalogue record for this book is available from the British Library.

ISBN 1 85775 368 2

Typeset by Advance Typesetting Ltd, Oxon.
Printed and bound by T.J. International Ltd.

Contents

Preface

This book has been designed to help all personnel working in primary healthcare to establish and maintain information systems that are necessary for effective working. The book is timed to coincide with the advent of primary care groups (PCGs), and therefore is written primarily for people involved with PCGs. However, it works from the practice level up, so it should (!) interest all members of the primary care team.

It tries to do at least six impossible things:

1 Talk about information in an interesting way.
2 Show how information can actually be useful.
3 Explain how to get you to love your computer.
4 Make Read Codes interesting.
5 Help practices to share meaningful information.
6 Make you smile while reading a book about information.

It includes references to incredibly unhip comedy series such as 'The Hitch Hiker's Guide to the Galaxy' (such as 'Why not round off this section by breakfast at Milliways, the Restaurant at the End of the Universe?').

The book assumes that you the reader are based in, or work with, a general practice. Each section includes exercises that generally require you to have access to a general practice. The book also uses nomenclature and examples from England and Wales, some of which may not apply to Scotland. However, Scottish readers should take comfort from the fact that sections such as that on MIQUEST(^{JB}) are of little relevance because the Scots are far ahead of south of the border in data sharing. Therefore Scottish readers should read on partly because there is much that is relevant, and partly for the smug self-satisfaction of knowing that once again, they are ahead of the game.

There is a Web site associated with this book. While it will be advantageous to have access to this, the book is designed to be largely accessible without Web access. For example, alternative sources are given for every resource identified as being available over the Web.

The book was fun to write. I hope it's fun to read.

Alan Gillies
July 1999

How to use the book

The book is organised into a series of sections. Broadly speaking, it is probably best if you read them in order. However, you may well find some material surplus to requirements. For example, Scottish readers do not need to know about MIQUEST(^{IB}). If you aren't into buying a new system, then Chapter 9 on procurement is irrelevant.

There are a number of common elements that recur throughout the book. Many of these have icons to help you spot them:

Once upon a time ...

There are a few fairy stories scattered through the book. As with all good fairy stories they begin with 'Once upon a time', but they contain serious messages.

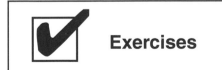 **Exercises**

Exercises generally occur at the end of chapters. They are designed to be carried out either by an individual or a group. They have a distinct output, generally in the form of a table. Model answers are given at the end of the book, but on the understanding that these are *model* answers. As most of the exercises relate to the reader's own experience, they may well have different detailed answers to the model answers given. The purpose of the model answers is to give an indication of the style of answer rather than the actual content.

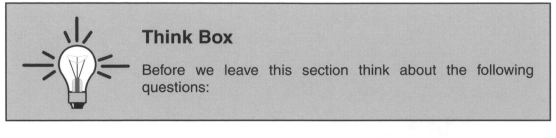

Think Boxes are designed to explore issues raised in the preceding chapters and exercises. They are designed for discussion, and would really benefit from the chance to discuss the answers with colleagues, either in a group situation or in a series of one-to-one encounters.

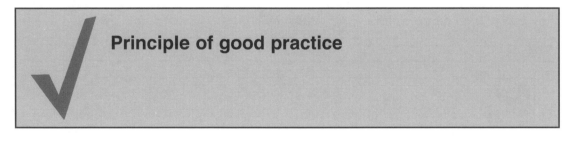

Key points are given at the end of each chapter to reinforce the key learning outcomes. They should not be used as a short cut, but rather as a check on knowledge gained. By the time you have completed the exercise, thought about the Think Box and reinforced key points, you should be ready to move on to the next section.

Principle of good practice

Principles of good practice are key practical issues. They represent an action that is good or best practice.

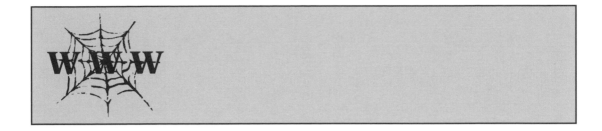

This is a World Wide Web link. It refers to resources accessible via the associated Web pages. However, it also tells you how to access the same resources without the use of the Web. Sadly, this may often involve a cost. These links refer to Appendices 1, 2 and 3 at the back of the book.

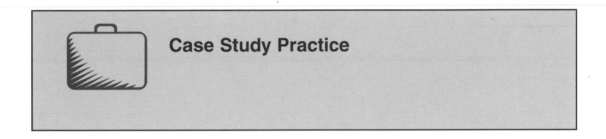

Case study practices are used to explore scenarios and illustrate teaching points. Generally, they are real practices, anonymised as a courtesy to the people involved.

10 points in a numbered list

1
2
...

The book also uses numbered lists extensively to summarise key points, contained within a shaded box.

(^{JB}) Finally, don't forget the jargon buster in Appendix 3. It contains explanation of a range of technical terms. A word included is identified by the (^{JB}) symbol in the text.

1

Why do we need information?

Once upon a time ...

... in a hot part of the world a long way away, there was a big country where someone caught a very nasty disease (actually, it was meningitis, but who wants to be pedantic in a fairy story?). The people were very poor and couldn't afford medicines. They certainly couldn't afford to waste their money recording how many people got ill. The disease was very infectious, and more and more people got ill and many of them died.

Now, one person from this country got ill but before he knew he was ill he went over the border into a little country next door. There he met lots of his friends and gave them the nasty disease. However, in this country was a man called the Epidemiologist. He noticed that too many people were getting ill and called his friends from the capital city to help him count how many people got ill. They didn't have any paper, so first they had to scrape around for some that was only written on one side. So they wrote on the back of envelopes, bills, anything they could find.

Soon they could show that too many people were ill and they sent a message to the Colonel in charge of the cavalry known as the World Health Organisation. The cavalry sent drugs and immunisations. The local people worked very hard and after many long days, they were able to stop any more people getting ill. Shortly after this the medical 'It's a Knockout' team turned up but were told that the game was over.

This may or not be a fairy story, but it's true that information is an important tool in healthcare today. As the health agenda switches from treating illness to keeping people healthy so information becomes more and more important.

And with the advent of PCGs, suddenly people not only have to have their own information, but they have to be able to swap information with other people.

This does make life a bit more complicated, although the Scots seem to have been doing it since the dawn of time (about 1989 in primary care computing terms).

Exercise 1

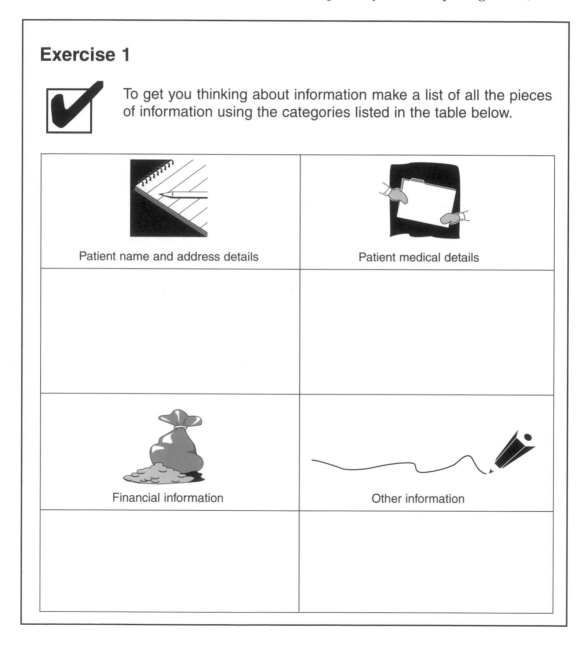

To get you thinking about information make a list of all the pieces of information using the categories listed in the table below.

Patient name and address details	Patient medical details
Financial information	Other information

The NHS has always used information. The classic information system in primary care has been a pile of Lloyd George envelopes. This may not seem very sexy as information systems go, but it served the NHS quite well for about 80 years.

Before we move on, let's think about this classic information system of the NHS.

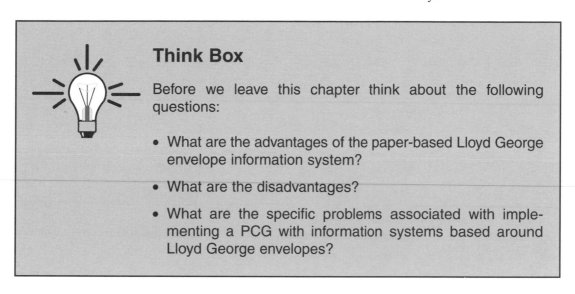

Think Box

Before we leave this chapter think about the following questions:

- What are the advantages of the paper-based Lloyd George envelope information system?

- What are the disadvantages?

- What are the specific problems associated with implementing a PCG with information systems based around Lloyd George envelopes?

Any replacement system must do better than this. In spite of the promise of new technology, many GP surgeries still depend on their old paper-based systems for much of their work. Only one in four practices in 1996 was using their computer systems within consultations.[1]

Primary care groups cannot work without good information, and therefore good information systems. The purpose of this handbook is to help you set up good systems to provide your PCG with high quality information. Only a small part of this task is about computers, so only a small part of this book is about them. First we must identify the information that we need.

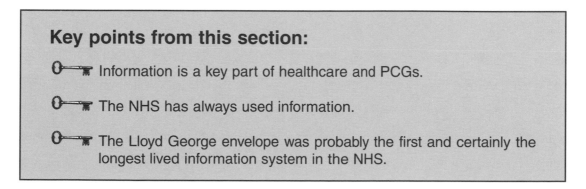

Key points from this section:

Information is a key part of healthcare and PCGs.

The NHS has always used information.

The Lloyd George envelope was probably the first and certainly the longest lived information system in the NHS.

---

[1] NHS Executive Computing Survey (1996) HMSO, London.

2

What information

do we need?

In any situation, the information needed is determined by the tasks that we are required to carry out.

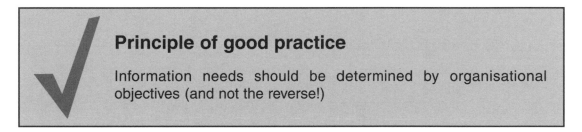

Principle of good practice

Information needs should be determined by organisational objectives (and not the reverse!)

According to the Government, PCGs will:

- contribute to the health authority's Health Improvement Programme (HIP) on health and healthcare, helping to ensure that this reflects the perspective of the local community and the experience of patients
- promote the health of the local population, working in partnership with other agencies
- commission health services for their populations from the relevant NHS trusts, within the framework of the HIP, ensuring quality and efficiency
- monitor performance against the service agreements they (or initially the health authority) have with NHS trusts
- develop primary care by joint working across practices; sharing skills; providing a forum for professional development, audit and peer review; assuring quality and developing the new approach to clinical governance; and influencing the deployment of resources for general practice locally. Local medical committees will have a key role in supporting this process

- better integrate primary and community health services and work more closely with social services on both planning and delivery. Services such as child health or rehabilitation, where responsibilities have been split within the health service and where liaison with local authorities is often poor, will particularly benefit.

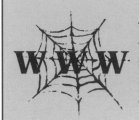 This comes from *The New NHS* White Paper of 1997. The full document is available on the World Wide Web and may be accessed via the Web site associated with this book. See Appendix 1 for details. A full paper reference is given in Appendix 2.

Translating this from Government-speak and compensating for political correctness, we can identify the following key tasks:

- health commissioning
- health promotion
- monitor performance
- clinical governance
- resource deployment among general practice
- work closely with other agencies.

In practice, these tasks cannot be separated from the provision of healthcare by general practice, so we must add the basic task of providing healthcare to patients on our list (it is easy to forget that this is what primary healthcare is all about really in the face of all these impressive sounding phrases!)

The Government has published a big document called the IM&T(*IB*) strategy.[2] In it, they suggest that all this should be based around an Electronic Health Record(*IB*). This is an example of a political BIG IDEA. As such it can be represented by a nice picture:

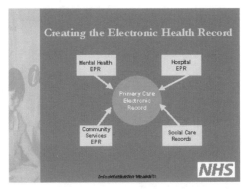

The electronic patient record according to the Department of Health, 1998.

---

[2]Department of Health (1998) *Information for Health: a new IM&T strategy.* HMSO, London.

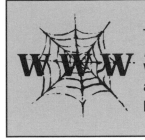

This comes from the New IM&T(^{JB}) strategy of 1998 entitled *Information for Health*. The full document is available on the World Wide Web and may be accessed via the Web site associated with this book. See Appendix 1 for details. A full paper reference is given in Appendix 2.

Unfortunately, the strategy is short on the detail of how to implement this pretty picture. So we shall go back to our rather more simple approach of looking at what information we need to do the things expected of a PCG and its component GP practices.

At its simplest, we need to know about our patients and about the activities undertaken to keep them healthy or restore them to health when they are ill. This means we have to keep information about patients and about procedures. In the previous chapter we identified two types of patient information: basic information about the patient, known as demographic data; and information about their medical history. Information about procedures was considered under two headings: financial and other. However, in these post-market days, we should perhaps simply refer to activity data, and consider information about the quantity and quality of activity.

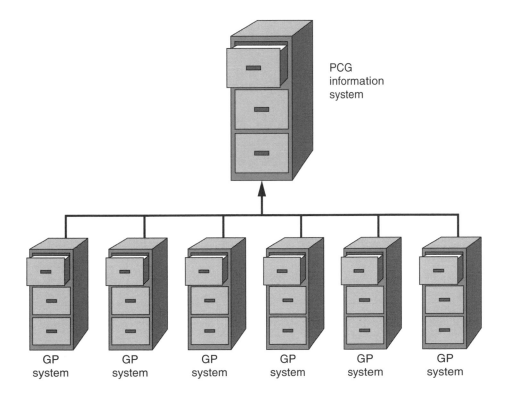

For our second exercise, we can use a modified version of the table in Exercise 1 to consider both the information requirements and the tasks that they support.

In practice, PCGs will largely use the information provided by GP systems. The information required by PCGs may be thought of as the collective information provided by the GP systems within the PCG with some additions to manage the collective roles of the PCG.

Exercise 2

 To establish what information we might need, make a list of all the pieces of information using the categories listed in the table below.

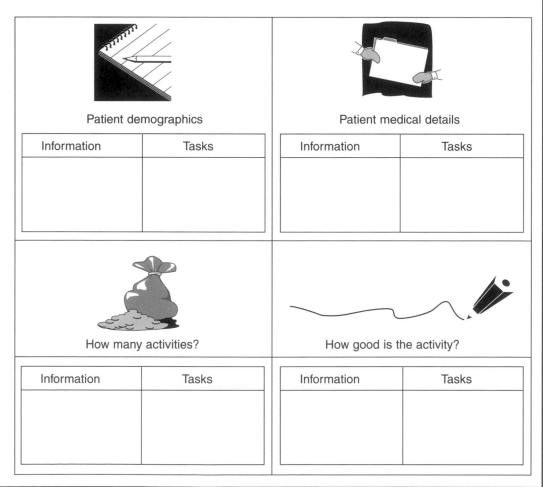

Patient demographics		Patient medical details	
Information	Tasks	Information	Tasks

How many activities?		How good is the activity?	
Information	Tasks	Information	Tasks

Therefore, we shall start defining our PCG information requirements by considering the information which should be available from component GP systems. After this we shall know what we need to add for our PCG system.

The Department of Health has defined what information should be stored in a GP system. This is known by the snappy title of 'The Rules for Accreditation 4'. (RFA4 for short) ([JB]). This is a model of a GP system that tells people what information systems for primary care should hold. We shall revisit this fount of knowledge for other goodies later. This model has six categories of information: practice, partners and staff, related organisations, patient registration, clinical record and drug database.

Of the four categories identified in Chapter 1 patient demographic details are known as patient registration and patient medical details are included in the clinical record.

However, the RFA4 model records some of its activity data within the clinical record, and separates prescribing activity as a distinct category known as 'prescribing and dispensing'. Just to confuse us, the RFA4 model also adds an extra category known as 'practice information'.

The RFA model is illustrated below.

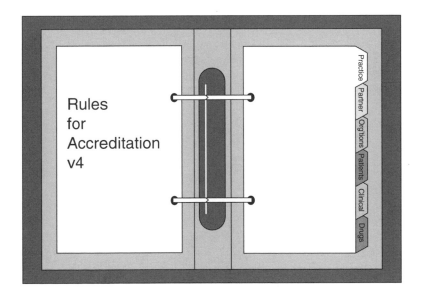

The full information requirements defined by RFA are shown in the following table.

Information specified by RFA4 for GP systems

Practice information	The practice	• Name and number of practice • Address(es) of surgery • Telephone and fax numbers • Fundholding practice number
	Partners and staff	• Name • Professional ID numbers • Role details • Contractual relationships with dates
	Related organisations	• Name and ID number • Address • Telephone and fax numbers • Contact details of key personnel
Patient information	Patient registration	• Surname, forename, title • DoB • Sex • Marital status • New NHS number (10-digit) • Old NHS number • Registration type • Registered home address • Previous or alternative address • Telephone contact number • Postcode • Responsible health authority • Registered GP • Usual GP • Dispensing status • Rural practice information • Date of removal
	Clinical record	• Medical, family and social history • Symptoms, signs and investigations • Diagnoses, sensitivities and problem
Prescribing and dispensing	Drug database	• All prescribable items • Interactions and contraindications • Doses and cautions • NHS price • NHS status and category

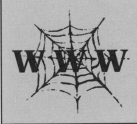 The complete *Rules for Accreditation([JB])* for GP Systems version 4 are to be found on the World Wide Web and may be accessed via the Web site associated with this book. See Appendix 1 for details. A full paper reference is given in Appendix 2.

The next step is to consider what we need to do to make use of this information in the context of PCGs, and what additional information is required. To do this, consider the six key tasks identified for PCGs:

- *Health commissioning* – to carry out effective health commissioning, PCGs need to match health needs of the population with health services provided by local hospitals and others. The health needs information comes from the GP clinical records. What is needed is information collected from all the GP systems covering the population. This information can and should be anonymous. We shall refer to this as our Patient Population Profile (PPP) and return to this in Chapter 4. However, we also need information on the availability, cost and quality of services from the supply side of what we used to call the NHS internal market.
- *Health promotion* – to plan effective health promotion, we need our PPP to identify the health needs in terms of health promotion. We also need to know what works. For this we need access to evidence and evidence-based resources such as clinical guidelines. The use of guidelines across the PCG should ensure consistent practice.
- *Monitoring performance* and *clinical governance* – both activities are concerned with using information to monitor the quality and quantity of activities. As such, the information required is contained within the clinical records and prescribing and dispensing sections of GP systems.
- *Resource deployment among general practice* – this is a PCG management function. However, the information required to assist in decision making is evidence both of health needs and practice activity. As such most of this can be drawn from the GP systems, the health needs coming from the patient records and the activity data coming from the patient records and the prescribing and dispensing sections.
- *Work closely with other agencies* – within the context of the new collaborative culture, it is necessary for PCGs to share information with other agencies both within the NHS and without. This can be a little tricky so we'll save this particular chestnut for later (Chapter 11).

Exercise 3

The above description depends on the PCGs having access to the information contained in the GP systems. What barriers are there to this?

To help you, the table below divides potential barriers into technical, legal and human.

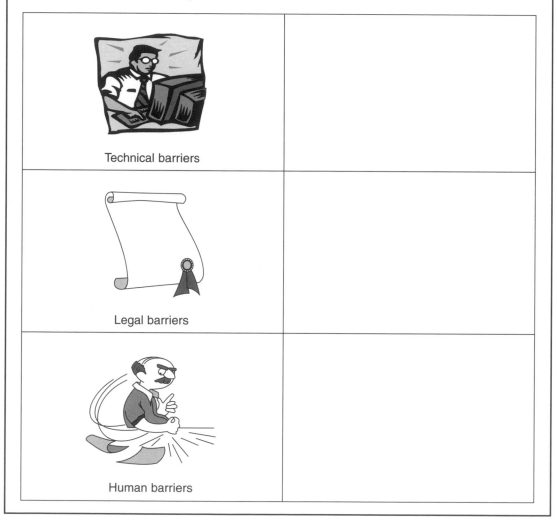

Technical barriers	
Legal barriers	
Human barriers	

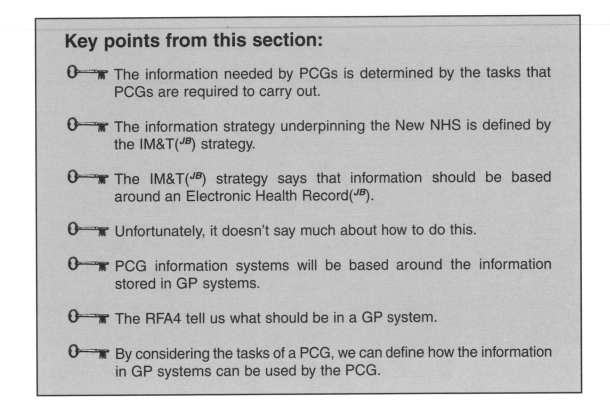

Think Box

Before we leave this section think about the following question:

- In this chapter, we introduced the idea of information systems for PCGs drawing on information from GP information systems. What changes could you make to the information and the way that it is stored by the PCG to reduce the barriers identified in Exercise 3?

Key points from this section:

⚷ The information needed by PCGs is determined by the tasks that PCGs are required to carry out.

⚷ The information strategy underpinning the New NHS is defined by the IM&T(JB) strategy.

⚷ The IM&T(JB) strategy says that information should be based around an Electronic Health Record(JB).

⚷ Unfortunately, it doesn't say much about how to do this.

⚷ PCG information systems will be based around the information stored in GP systems.

⚷ The RFA4 tell us what should be in a GP system.

⚷ By considering the tasks of a PCG, we can define how the information in GP systems can be used by the PCG.

3

You really mean computers, don't you?

So far we have managed to avoid the c******* word (well almost, we've mentioned it twice, in fact). Maybe you're getting cross because you thought this book was going to be about computers and you thought I was joking in Chapter 1 (what do you mean you didn't read it because it was only an introduction?). OK, for any techies among you here goes … a section on computers!

The trouble with computers in the NHS is too often they are like elephants([JB]) …

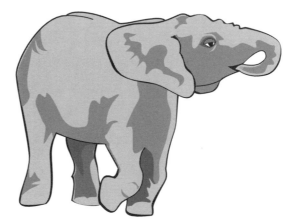

… you feed a lot of stuff in, most of it disappears into the elephant's innards and all that you get out is a pile of dung!

The history of the NHS and IT is not a happy one. Ask the Secretary of State: 'Up to now the use of IT in the NHS has not been a success story. Far from it. Lots of money has been wasted. Some important data has not been collected and used. Other data has been collected but not used …'

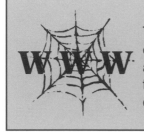

This comes from the Foreword of the New IM&T(^{JB}) strategy of 1998 entitled *Information for Health*. The full document is available on the World Wide Web and may be accessed via the Web site associated with this book. See Appendix 1 for details. A full paper reference is given in Appendix 2.

Here's my list of some of the reasons why IT hasn't been a success.

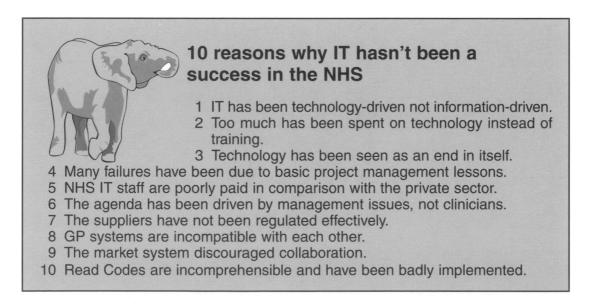

10 reasons why IT hasn't been a success in the NHS

1 IT has been technology-driven not information-driven.
2 Too much has been spent on technology instead of training.
3 Technology has been seen as an end in itself.
4 Many failures have been due to basic project management lessons.
5 NHS IT staff are poorly paid in comparison with the private sector.
6 The agenda has been driven by management issues, not clinicians.
7 The suppliers have not been regulated effectively.
8 GP systems are incompatible with each other.
9 The market system discouraged collaboration.
10 Read Codes are incomprehensible and have been badly implemented.

However, it really doesn't have to be like this. Computers can actually make life easier (no, honestly, I mean it!). You do, however, need to do things a bit differently.

To get you started, there are at least ten good things you can do to help improve things. Please note that buying a new computer doesn't figure in my top ten, but I guess if you don't have one, maybe it should!

These positive principles will guide the rest of the book. Computers can actually be a help. However, state-of-the-art technology is not a critical success factor. Consider two practices with successful computer systems, both of which have featured as examples of best practice in information management. The first has invested heavily in technology, and made very effective use of that technology. Our second practice provides a contrast in technology but an equally effective information solution.

---

10 ways to improve the chances of success with IT!

1 Start by considering information needs, not technology.
2 Invest heavily in training for clinicians as well as IT staff.
3 Involve clinicians in all IT decisions.
4 Technology is a means to an end.
5 Use proper project management techniques.
6 Use the best IT staff you can.
7 Ensure that the IT solution delivers better patient care and clinical benefits.
8 Ensure that the suppliers deliver what's promised.
9 Adopt recommended solutions across the PCG to minimise compatibility problems.
10 Adopt a PCG-wide coding policy.

Case Study Practice 1

Practice 1 is a practice of 10 500 patients with four doctors, based in a market town, surrounded by a rural area. The catchment area covers 100 square miles. The practice is extremely innovative. It was a first wave fundholding practice and has been computerised since 1987.

It is currently using a computer system launched in 1997, with state-of-the-art features and a graphical user interface. The practice is completely paperless except for consultations remote from the surgery, which are recorded on paper forms and then entered by the physicians on their return.

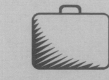

Case Study Practice 1 *continued*

The practice has developed largely autonomously. It pioneered electronic links for lab results by moving its contract away from their NHS provider to a private company. The practice shows a mature use of its information system. In terms of maximising the benefits from the system, the only two omissions are in the area of external electronic links and the use of paper forms for remote data collection. The gap in external links will largely be addressed by the advent of NHSNet([JB]). For remote data entry, a laptop has been introduced, but the practice is currently evaluating its options. Hand-held computers were piloted a year or so ago, but withdrawn due to inadequate technology. This may have changed with the advent of the latest devices.

Case Study Practice 2

Practice 2 is a large practice with six doctors, based in a deprived urban area. The practice is based in a local health centre and its patients nearly all live within 3 miles of the practice. The practice is extremely innovative. It was a first wave fundholding practice and has been computerised since 1987.

It is still using its original computer system, which lacks many of the features of the latest systems and has an exclusively text-based interface.

However, the practice has tailored the system extensively to meet its needs, enabling it to make extensive use of computerised guidelines and protocols within consultations. The system is used extensively for real-time audits.

Other innovations include electronic patient information systems within the surgery. The effort and resource invested in tailoring the system acts as a significant disincentive to upgrading. However, the quality of the information provided by the current system is very impressive.

The key point from these examples is that there are good information systems based around limited technology, and bad information systems based around advanced technology. Therefore we shall now forget about computers for a while longer.

Exercise 4

Use the table below to assess the digestive habits of your ~~elephant~~ computer system. Delete any information that you don't collect from the left-hand column and any from the right that doesn't come out again.

Information in	Information out
• Name and number of practice	• Name and number of practice
• Address(es) of surgery	• Address(es) of surgery
• Telephone and fax numbers	• Telephone and fax numbers
• Fundholding practice number	• Fundholding practice number*
• Name	• Name
• Professional ID numbers	• Professional ID numbers
• Role details	• Role details
• Contractual relationships with dates	• Contractual relationships with dates
• Surname, Forename, Title	• Surname, Forename, Title
• DoB	• DoB
• Sex	• Sex
• Marital status	• Marital status
• New NHS number (10-digit)	• New NHS number (10-digit)
• Old NHS number	• Old NHS number
• Registration type	• Registration type
• Registered home address	• Registered home address
• Previous or alternative address	• Previous or alternative address
• Telephone contact number	• Telephone contact number
• Postcode	• Postcode
• Responsible health authority	• Responsible health authority
• Registered GP	• Registered GP
• Usual GP	• Usual GP
• Dispensing status	• Dispensing status
• Rural practice information	• Rural practice information
• Date of removal	• Date of removal
• Medical, family and social history	• Medical, family and social history
• Symptoms, signs and investigations	• Symptoms, signs and investigations
• Diagnoses, sensitivities and problem	• Diagnoses, sensitivities and problem
• All prescribable items	• All prescribable items
• Interactions and contraindications	• Interactions and contraindications
• Doses and cautions	• Doses and cautions
• NHS price	• NHS price
• NHS status and category	• NHS status and category

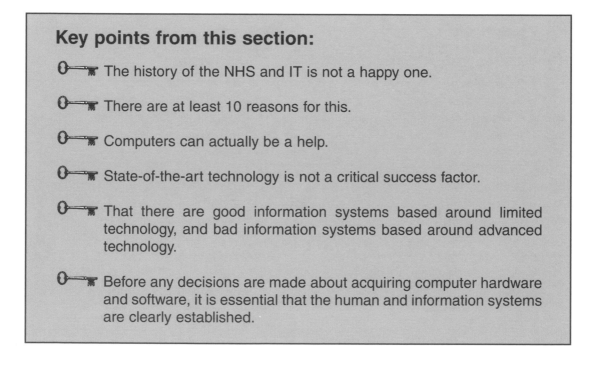

Think Box

Before we leave this section think about the following question:

• The Secretary of State said 'Some important data has not been collected and used. Other data has been collected but not used ...'. What examples can you give from your own work of:

(a) important data which has not been collected?

(b) other data which has been collected but not used?

Key points from this section:

The history of the NHS and IT is not a happy one.

There are at least 10 reasons for this.

Computers can actually be a help.

State-of-the-art technology is not a critical success factor.

That there are good information systems based around limited technology, and bad information systems based around advanced technology.

Before any decisions are made about acquiring computer hardware and software, it is essential that the human and information systems are clearly established.

4

Thinking about information in your PCG

So far we have identified in piecemeal fashion the bits of information that we need to run the PCG. We have also identified the fact that much of this information exists in the GP systems of the practices that make up the group.

In this chapter we shall identify the information required by the PCG and where it will come from. If we return to our picture of the PCG information system as feeding from the GP systems, we can identify where the different information types will be stored.

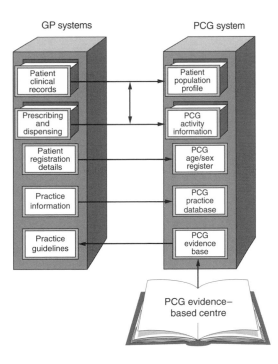

We have previously identified two key types of information for the PCG, concerning patient and activity information.

The patient information is represented in the PPP. This is a collation of the clinical records from all the GP systems. However, as the patient registration details are held separately, this ensures that the data held at PCG level are population-based. By anonymising data in this way, the confidentiality of patient records is maintained. The purposes for which this information is used, health commissioning, health promotion, performance monitoring and clinical governance and epidemiological research, do not require identification of individual patients.

Principle of good practice

Information should only be stored and distributed on a 'need to know' basis.

For cross reference back to GP systems, a patient identifier may be added. This should be meaningless to the PCG, but allow GPs to identify their own patients where required. In practice the PPP should include information about prescribing, as this forms part of the clinical record and may be required for the above purposes.

The second type of information required at the PCG level is information about the quality and quantity of activity for performance monitoring and clinical governance purposes. In practice, this information is stored in both the clinical record and prescribing and dispensing sections of our conceptual GP system. However, we shall see later that in practice the Electronic Health Record(^{JB}) used to store the information in practice in GP systems links prescribing to patient records, so this is not a practical problem.

To operate at the higher levels of activity, the PCG will need to keep a record of the patients registered, in the form of an age/sex register storing basic demographic information in patient-identifiable form. The PCG will also need to keep a record of practice information, including employee information and other practice information held within the GP system.

Finally, to meet the demands of the delivery of evidence-based healthcare and the requirement to validate practice for clinical governance, the PCG will need access to evidence. Many PCGs are seeking to establish their own evidence-based centres to provide this information. These will in turn feed off other regional and national initiatives.

The best way to distribute the evidence is in the form of computer-based guidelines and protocols distributed to individual practices.

It should be stressed that this is a conceptual model of information systems. The information does not have to be physically located within the PCG. For example, the information within GP systems can remain there, provided that the PCG can have access to the information. In the days of an NHS-wide network, PCGs should not be creating duplicate information sets, but accessing GP systems as required.

In the next chapter, we shall see how this might be achieved.

Exercise 5

At present, and in the early days of PCGs, the functions identified as belonging to the PCG are carried out by the health authority. These systems are the starting point for the PCG systems of the future. Identify for yourself which of the functions described are currently supported by your health authority and their information systems. Also find out how (or if) these systems link to general practice. Remember the systems may be paper-based, as well as computerised.

Health authority systems	Links to GP systems

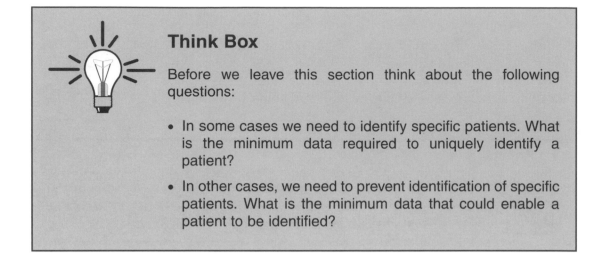

Think Box

Before we leave this section think about the following questions:

- In some cases we need to identify specific patients. What is the minimum data required to uniquely identify a patient?
- In other cases, we need to prevent identification of specific patients. What is the minimum data that could enable a patient to be identified?

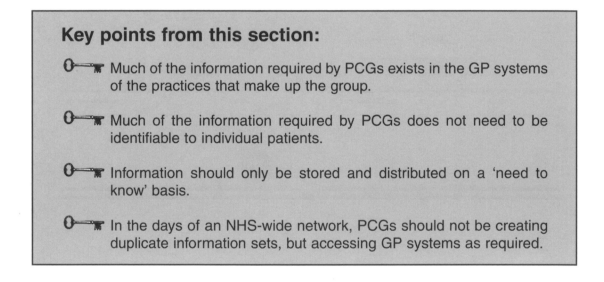

Key points from this section:

Much of the information required by PCGs exists in the GP systems of the practices that make up the group.

Much of the information required by PCGs does not need to be identifiable to individual patients.

Information should only be stored and distributed on a 'need to know' basis.

In the days of an NHS-wide network, PCGs should not be creating duplicate information sets, but accessing GP systems as required.

5

Why you need those horrible computers

Ah! You knew we'd get back to computers before too long, didn't you. We need computers because our paper-based systems simply cannot provide adequate information to support the information needs of a large modern practice let alone a PCG. However, computers are simply a means to an end to deliver the information system we need. On their own, they cannot solve our problems. If you don't know how to get from London to Manchester, then having a fast car is as likely to take you away from Manchester as towards it. Worse, if you set off in the wrong direction, the faster the car, the further away it will take you in a given period of time. Computers are fast cars compared with Lloyd George envelopes, which are more like push bikes, but you can still head off hurtling towards the English Channel, if you don't know where you're going.

The purpose of this chapter is to understand better what computers can and cannot do, so that we can use them appropriately and effectively to achieve the goals of better healthcare delivery and management.

Let's first consider what computers are good at.

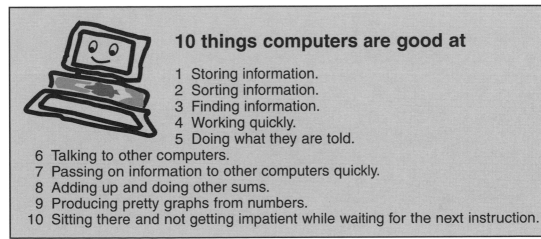

10 things computers are good at

1 Storing information.
2 Sorting information.
3 Finding information.
4 Working quickly.
5 Doing what they are told.
6 Talking to other computers.
7 Passing on information to other computers quickly.
8 Adding up and doing other sums.
9 Producing pretty graphs from numbers.
10 Sitting there and not getting impatient while waiting for the next instruction.

But equally, there are things that computers are bad at; ten of these are listed below. The best way to think about this is to consider the computer as a member of your team, with particular strengths and weaknesses. As in any team situation good practice requires that you play to the computer's strengths and compensate for its weaknesses. Very often, problems are caused by people's false expectations of their computer systems.

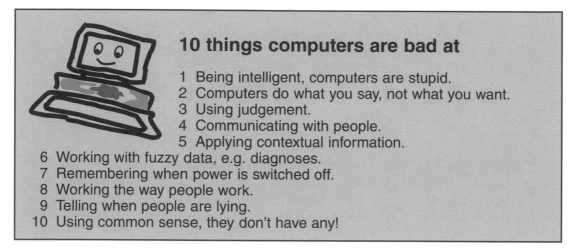

10 things computers are bad at

1 Being intelligent, computers are stupid.
2 Computers do what you say, not what you want.
3 Using judgement.
4 Communicating with people.
5 Applying contextual information.
6 Working with fuzzy data, e.g. diagnoses.
7 Remembering when power is switched off.
8 Working the way people work.
9 Telling when people are lying.
10 Using common sense, they don't have any!

Principle of good practice

Understand the strengths and weaknesses of your computer and play to its strengths.

Computers treat information very literally. To you, 'heart attack' and 'myocardial infarction' may be similar, but to the computer they are not. Everything that you want the computer to know, it has to be told. For example, if you told the computer any of the following:

- the patient is –70 years old
- the patient is 700 years old
- the patient is older than his parents
- the patient was born tomorrow

the computer will only query these statements if given a specific instruction so to do. Computers work best when information is precise and unambiguous. The problem is that, in healthcare, information rarely is.

In the next chapter, we shall see the major implication of using computers. To make effective use of computers, it is essential to represent information in a computer-friendly form. Unfortunately, this is not a people-friendly form. We must bite the bullet and look at Read Codes.

Exercise 6

In this exercise, we want to look at the implications of the strengths and weaknesses of computers for their use in PCGs.

In the following table, think of an instance and the implication where each strength and weakness affects the management and delivery of healthcare within the PCG. One example is done to help you.

Strength/Weakness	Instance	Implication
✔ Storing information ✔ Sorting information ✔ Finding information ✔ Working quickly ✔ Doing what they are told ✔ Talking to other computers ✔ Passing on information to other computers quickly ✔ Adding up and doing other sums ✔ Producing pretty graphs from numbers ✔ Sitting there and not getting impatient while waiting for the next instruction ✘ Not being intelligent ✘ Computers do what you say, not what you want ✘ They don't use judgement ✘ Bad at communicating with people ✘ Applying contextual information ✘ Working with fuzzy data, e.g. diagnoses ✘ Remembering when power is switched off ✘ Working the way people work ✘ Telling when people are lying ✘ Using common sense, they don't have any!	Consultation	Can find patient record

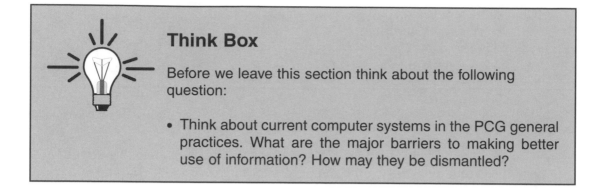

Think Box

Before we leave this section think about the following question:

- Think about current computer systems in the PCG general practices. What are the major barriers to making better use of information? How may they be dismantled?

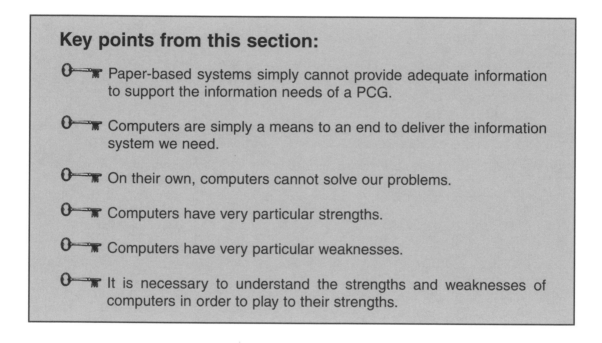

Key points from this section:

🔑 Paper-based systems simply cannot provide adequate information to support the information needs of a PCG.

🔑 Computers are simply a means to an end to deliver the information system we need.

🔑 On their own, computers cannot solve our problems.

🔑 Computers have very particular strengths.

🔑 Computers have very particular weaknesses.

🔑 It is necessary to understand the strengths and weaknesses of computers in order to play to their strengths.

6

Why you need those even more horrible Read Codes

Have you ever seen a Read Code? Do you know what one is?

In the overall scale of things, Read Codes are not attractive objects. They do not have ascetic beauty, mathematical elegance or even basic comprehensibility.

It is therefore unfortunate that Read Codes are probably the second most important thing to get right about your information solution for your PCG (the first being the people side of things). So the first job must be to explain why coding is important and why Read Codes are the only viable codes to use for your PCG. It is perhaps too much to hope that you should ever come to love Read Codes, and frankly if you do, then the best advice is either to get a life or seek professional counselling.

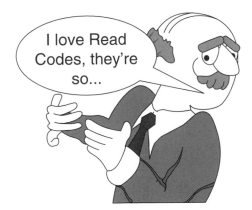

People use natural language to communicate and to describe things. It has the advantage of being known to everyone, very flexible, able to express shades of opinion and fuzziness. However, from the computer's point of view it is complex, inconsistent and requires a great deal of contextual information to interpret ambiguities. As we have seen, computers can process information quickly, but only if it is clear and unambiguous.

Just as human language has evolved to meet our information processing needs, so systems have evolved to meet the information processing needs of computers. Coding systems meet a need to describe the world of healthcare in concise and unambiguous ways.

The first major coding systems were used to describe diseases within epidemiology. Schemes of this type are ICD-9 and ICD-10[IB]. They provide a code made up of letters and numbers for just about every disease on the planet. They form a kind of Esperanto for epidemiologists. But disease coding is inadequate for primary care. And so it's time for another fairy story.

Once upon a time ...

… there was a doctor who lived in a town famous for producing books named after red and black insects. One day he worked out that what the world really needed was a system which could describe all of general practice, hitherto only describable in nice human terms such as 'the common cold', 'a bad back', in completely incomprehensible, apparently random sets of letters and numbers such as G3011. What is even more remarkable is that he (allegedly) worked out that this might be worth a lot of money because these nasty computer thingies actually liked incomprehensible sets of letters and numbers.

And so he started to write these codes. They began as two-character codes and covered a simple list of symptoms, diagnoses, procedures and drugs. However, people began to get the hang of things, so it wasn't long before he needed to expand to three-character and four-character codes to confuse people again. Soon he had to come with a new name, so he called his codes the 4-byte set.

By now, people were really catching on, so he invented a whole new version called Version 2. But as it was really quite easy to understand that this was just a new version, he then invented another version and, by now running out of ways to confuse people, he called it Version 3.

By now other doctors were starting to get envious so they started to allege that this had all made him a lot of money. However, this was found not to be the case by an enquiry, and so the good doctor was allowed to go inventing even more confusing codes.

Of course, the fairy story is just that. Read Codes are, however, crucial to primary healthcare and to PCGs. First, we shall see five reasons why coding is essential and then second, why Read Codes are the only suitable coding systems for PCGs.

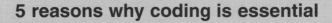

5 reasons why coding is essential

1 Codes provide unambiguous information suitable for computer processing.
2 Codes allow standard morbidity data to be collected across a PCG population.
3 Codes allow the definition and implementation of standard clinical guidelines and protocols across the practices of a PCG.
4 Codes allow the collection of standard data sets for performance monitoring and clinical governance.
5 Coding facilitates comparison between and within PCGs.

5 reasons why Read Codes are essential

1 Read Codes cover the whole remit of primary care and much beyond primary care. My favourite is 'accidental poisoning occurring in an opera house'.
2 Read Codes are hierarchical, allowing different levels of detail in different situations.
3 Read Codes are updated every 3 months (drugs every month).
4 Read Codes can be cross referenced to all other major systems, e.g. ICD, OPCS, BNF, ATC, etc.
5 Coding only works if everyone talks the same language. Read Codes are the UK NHS standard, therefore all other reasons are redundant.

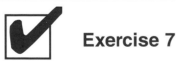

Exercise 7

Two (almost!) fun things to do with Read Codes:

1 Find an even more obscure code than 'accidental poisoning occurring in an opera house'.

2 Complete the slogan 'I love Read Codes because they're so …' in not more than 15 words.

In practice, the Read Codes are intended to cover the following areas:

- diseases
- occupations
- history/symptoms
- examinations/signs
- diagnostic procedures
- radiology/diagnostic imaging
- preventive procedures
- operative procedures
- other therapeutic procedures
- administration
- drugs/appliances.

So for the uninitiated, what do Read Codes look like? They are generally described as being 'hierarchical' in nature. This means that the more letters or numbers you add the more precise the code becomes.

Consider, for example, ischaemic heart disease. We shall use version 2 to illustrate it because it is still the most commonly used form of Read Codes. In Read Code Speak, a simple letter 'G' represents the circulatory system. Add a '3' to make a 'G3' code and we get to a code for ischaemic heart disease. Add more numbers and we get more detail. If we carry on adding more numbers to our example it goes as follows:

Circulatory system	G
Ischaemic heart disease	G3
Acute myocardial infarction	G30
Anterior acute myocardial infarction	G301
Acute anteroseptal myocardial infarction	G3011

These may look pretty daunting, but there are important things that may make Read Codes less intimidating.

First, Read Codes include 'synonyms' for clinical terminology. Thus within the coding system, while each concept has a preferred term, many also have synonymous terms. In our case, for example, 'G30' represents 'acute myocardial infarction', which is known as the preferred term, but this concept may also be described as 'heart attack', 'acute MI' or 'MI' (among others). These terms are provided as synonyms and all have the same code as 'acute myocardial infarction' (G30).

Second, much of the Read Code terminology can, once defined, be hidden inside the computer system. Thus the system will automatically enter a G30 code when a doctor pulls any of the above terms off a list of clinical diagnoses on his or her computer screen.

The really important issue for PCGs is to set up all the practice information systems within their group to do the following.

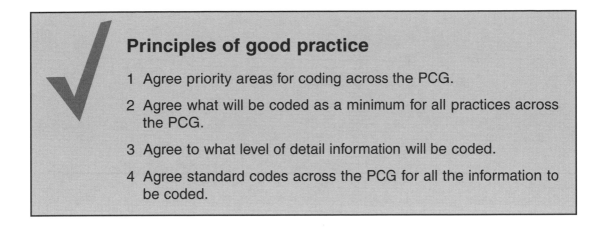

Principles of good practice

1 Agree priority areas for coding across the PCG.

2 Agree what will be coded as a minimum for all practices across the PCG.

3 Agree to what level of detail information will be coded.

4 Agree standard codes across the PCG for all the information to be coded.

Fortunately, you don't have to make all these decisions on your own. There is a national project set up to assist with the **C**ollection of **H**ealth **D**ata in **G**eneral **P**ractice (hence its name, CHDGP).

They have a Web site and from it you can download a very useful document known as the Co-ordinator's Handbook.

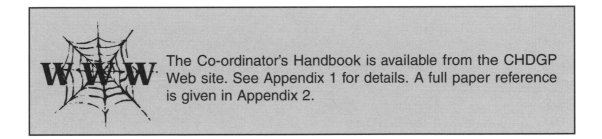

The Co-ordinator's Handbook is available from the CHDGP Web site. See Appendix 1 for details. A full paper reference is given in Appendix 2.

For example, the CHDGP Handbook will tell you that the national project is focused around morbidity data in six key areas, linked closely to national health promotion targets:

- heart disease and related conditions
- cerebrovascular disease and related conditions
- hypertension
- diabetes
- asthma
- severe mental illness (psychoses and similar conditions).

The Handbook provides guidelines which should form the basis of any PCG data collection initiative.

CHDGP Guidelines for data collection

1 Whenever a patient presents with a morbidity (or morbidities) from the core data set, a recording of the appropriate code or codes is made to denote this encounter. The words appropriate code (or codes) refer to the morbidity; if other investigations are made which are referred to in the core data set, these are also to be recorded.

2 The relevant risk factors will also be recorded, again as appropriate.

3 Any numerical values associated with the code, such as BP readings, should also be recorded.

4 The entry should be dated with the date on which the encounter took place.

5 The entry should be attributed to the clinician with whom the encounter took place.

6 The nature of the episode of the morbidity to which the encounter relates should be recorded.

The Handbook provides lots of useful advice on how to maximise the quality of the data and is proof that there really are useful resources to be had for free from the Internet (providing you buy this book first to tell you where to look!).

Having established the coding policy for your PCG, which details the codes to be collected and the manner in which they are to be collected, it is then necessary to collect the coded information from the constituent practices. There are two key types of barriers here, technical and professional.

The technical barriers are based on the fact that all the major GP computer systems are incompatible and will not talk to each other. This is a major reason why it was suggested earlier that your PCG should try to focus on a limited number of systems.

The professional barriers relate to concerns over data protection and confidentiality. There are often very genuine concerns on the part of professionals about the sharing of sensitive personal clinical information.

The proposed solution to these twin problems is MIQUEST(^{JB}). MIQUEST(^{JB}) is a combination of a software tool to overcome the technical barriers and a set of procedural guidelines to allay fears over confidentiality.

The technical part of MIQUEST(^{JB}) is a query language and an interpreter. The query language is, funnily enough, a language in which you write queries. An example of query would be 'How many patients have had a heart attack in the last year?'.

Schematically, we can think of MIQUEST(*IB*) as below:

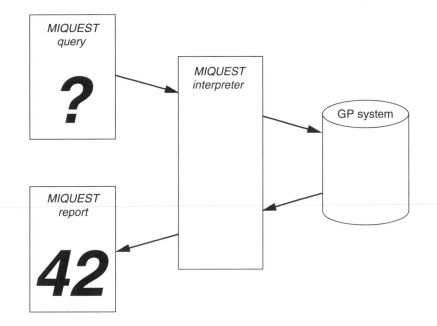

A query is written the MIQUEST(*IB*) query language asking: 'How many heart attacks occurred among your patients between 01/01/98 and 31/12/98?'.

The MIQUEST(*IB*) interpreter is able to translate the query written in MIQUEST(*IB*) speak into EMIS speak or MEDITEL speak, or whatever form the GP system requires. This causes the GP system to search its patient records to find how many G30 Read Codes are recorded with dates in 1998.

It then sends the number to the MIQUEST(*IB*) interpreter, which produces a report saying there were 42 cases during 1998. Now, MIQUEST(*IB*) may not be able to come up with the answer to Life, the Universe and Everything (42).[3] However, it is at least an attempt to deal with data collection from incompatible systems.

The second part of MIQUEST(*IB*) is the MIQUEST(*IB*) data collection protocols. These contain full data security and confidentiality safeguards.

---

[3]In *The Hitch Hiker's Guide to The Galaxy* (Pan Books, 1978), Deep Thought claims that 42 is the answer to the ultimate question of Life, the Universe and Everything. Apologies to younger readers!

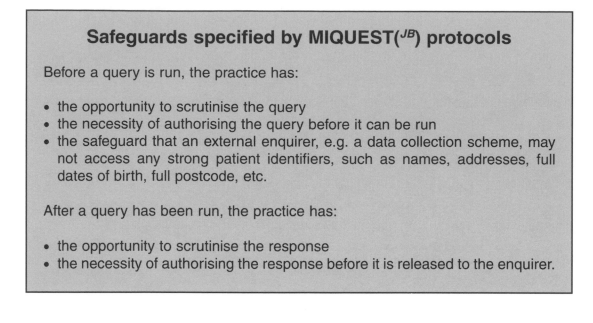

Safeguards specified by MIQUEST(^{JB}) protocols

Before a query is run, the practice has:

- the opportunity to scrutinise the query
- the necessity of authorising the query before it can be run
- the safeguard that an external enquirer, e.g. a data collection scheme, may not access any strong patient identifiers, such as names, addresses, full dates of birth, full postcode, etc.

After a query has been run, the practice has:

- the opportunity to scrutinise the response
- the necessity of authorising the response before it is released to the enquirer.

In practice, the author believes that MIQUEST(^{JB}) is a technically complex solution brought about as a response to bad historical planning and the victory of ideology over common sense. This wouldn't matter if there weren't some unfortunate consequences for PCGs. The problems generally lie with the MIQUEST(^{JB}) interpreter.

Potential problems for PCGs with MIQUEST(^{JB})

- Each system requires its own interpreter.
- The interpreters must be written by the suppliers.
- The PCG needs an interpreter for every type of system within its group.
- Early interpreters proved unreliable.
- Some companies have been lukewarm in their support for MIQUEST(^{JB}), e.g. Meditel have, as far as I am aware, refused to develop one for their old Medical system in favour of the newer System 6000.

The plans for version 5 (due to be launched in October 1999, with conformant systems appearing in 2000) of the Rules for Accreditation(^{JB}) of GP systems, to which suppliers must conform if they wish to attract funding for GP systems, show that MIQUEST(^{JB}) compatibility will be a requirement. However, this will not deal with older systems which are already in place. There is no incentive for suppliers to develop interpreters for these systems.

In cases such as these, it will be necessary for the PCG to write special queries to interrogate those systems which cannot be accessed by MIQUEST(^{JB}). These queries must be written with great care to ensure compatibility with the MIQUEST(^{JB}) queries.

On the next two pages there is a special section for those who feel cheated by the lack of technical gobbledygook in the book so far. I have included a sample MIQUEST(^{JB}) query and report. This query will provide age and sex data for a target population. Note the report starts by reiterating the query.

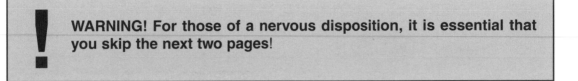

WARNING! For those of a nervous disposition, it is essential that you skip the next two pages!

Sample MIQUEST(^{JB}) Query

```
"*QRY_WDATE,19971007,07/10/1997"
"*QRY_SDATE,19971007,07/10/1997"
"*QRY_ORDER,001"
"*QRY_TITLE,AGESEX,Age sex breakdown for practice"
"*ENQ_RSPID,UNKNOWN,Unknown respondent"
"*QRY_MEDIA,D,Disk"
"*QRY_AGREE,UNKNOWN,Unknown agreement"
"*QRY_SETID,READ5AGE,Emis Read 5 standard query set – age sex"
"*ENQ_IDENT,CHDGP,Countyshire Scheme Coordinator"
"DEFINE AGE AS @YEARS(""11/05/1998"",DATE_OF_BIRTH)"
ANALYSE
"GROUPED_BY SEX (""M"";""F"")"
"AND AGE (""0""-""4"";""5""-""9"";""10""-""14"";""15""-""19"";""20""-""24"";""25""-
""29"";""30""-""34""\"
";""35""-""39"";""40""-""44"";""45""-""49"";""50""-""54"";""55""-""59"";""60""-""64"";""65""-
""69"";""70""\"
"-""74"";""75""-""79"";""80""-""84"";""85""-""89"";""90""-""94"";""95""-""99"";""100""-
""104"";""105""\"
"-""109"")"
FROM PATIENTS
```

Sample MIQUEST(^{JB}) Report

```
*QRY_WDATE,19971007,07/10/97
"
*QRY_SDATE,19980616,16/06/98
"*QRY_ORDER,1,
*QRY_TITLE,AGESEX,Age sex breakdown for practice
*ENQ_RSPID,NWL02,
*QRY_MEDIA,D,Disk
*QRY_AGREE,SIP,Sharing Information in Primary
*QRY_SETID,READ5AGE,Emis Read 5 standard query set – age sex
*ENQ_IDENT,DCM,Nina Kumari
"DEFINE AGE AS @YEARS(""11/05/1998""",DATE_OF_BIRTH),
ANALYSE,,
"GROUPED_BY SEX (""M"""";""F""")",,
#M is the SEX for Male,,
#F is the SEX for Female,,
"AND AGE (""0""-""4"";""5""-""9"";""10""-""14"";""15""-""19"";""20""-""24"";""25""-
""29"";""30""-""34"";""35""-""39"";""40""-""44"";""45""-""49"";""50""-""54"";""55""-
""59"";""60""-""64"";""65""-""69"";""70""-""74"";""75""-""79"";""80""-""84"";""85""-
""89"";""90""-""94"";""95""-""99"";""100""-""104"";""105""-""109""")",,
FROM PATIENTS,,

*RSP_IDENT,P81748,
*RSP_AUTHR,,
*RSP_RDATE,19980627,1307
&0,ANALYSE,2
SEX,AGE,
F,0-4,191
F,05-Sep,213
F,Oct-14,193
F,15-19,150
F,20-24,143
F,25-29,261
F,30-34,284
F,35-39,223
F,40-44,201
F,45-49,172
F,50-54,191
F,55-59,164
F,60-64,153
F,65-69,147
F,70-74,144
```

Sample MIQUEST(^{JB}) Report *continued*

```
F,75-79,120
F,80-84,82
F,85-89,58
F,90-94,18
F,95-99,4
F,100-104,1
F,105-109,0
M,0-4,228
M,05-Sep,228
M,Oct-14,218
M,15-19,146
M,20-24,133
M,25-29,225
M,30-34,281
M,35-39,276
M,40-44,181
M,45-49,191
M,50-54,178
M,55-59,162
M,60-64,145
M,65-69,114
M,70-74,101
M,75-79,77
M,80-84,35
M,85-89,12
M,90-94,1
M,95-99,1
M,100-104,0
M,105-109,0
```

Exercise 8

Use the table below to identify the current coding policy of your organisation. If your own does no coding ask around the other members of your PCG to see what they are doing.

Clinical areas covered	Clinical terms identified	Read Codes

Exercise 9

 Use the table below to identify a potential future coding policy for your PCG. You would be best advised to look at the Think Box for this section before tackling this exercise.

Clinical areas to be covered	Clinical terms identified	Read Codes

Think Box

Before we leave this section think about the following question:

Which clinical areas are of local interest and might be suitable for investigation alongside those suggested by the National CHDGP project?

Key points from this section:

- Read Codes are probably the second most important thing to get right about your information solution for your PCG.

- Computers can process information quickly, but only if it is clear and unambiguous.

- Coding systems meet a need to describe the world of healthcare in concise and unambiguous ways.

- Coding is essential.

- Read Codes are essential.

- Much of the Read Code terminology can be hidden inside the computer system once defined.

- It is essential for the PCG to define a coding policy.

- There are two key types of barriers to data collection, technical and professional.

- MIQUEST([JB]) addresses these problems.

- MIQUEST([JB]) is not perfect.

- It will be necessary for the PCG to write special queries to interrogate those systems which cannot be accessed by MIQUEST([JB]).

7

Where you are now

The starting point for implementing your new information system across the PCG is to carry out an audit of the general practices within your group. However, you are not starting from scratch. The health authority should already hold the basic practice information.

This will include the following information about the practice itself:

- name and number of practice
- address(es) of surgery
- telephone and fax numbers
- fundholding practice number (where applicable).

The following about the partners and staff:

- name
- professional ID numbers
- role details
- contractual relationships with dates.

The following about related organisations:

- name and ID number
- address
- telephone and fax numbers
- contact details of key personnel.

And hopefully the following about the practice information system:

- supplier
- version
- coding system and version.

The first step in making progress is to establish how developed the practices are in terms of their use of information. The author has developed a model for such a purpose, and we will use it to establish development plans for every practice in order to enable them to contribute to the PCG information system.

The model is known as the GPIMM, which stands for the General Practice Information Maturity Model.

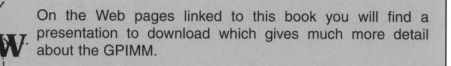

On the Web pages linked to this book you will find a presentation to download which gives much more detail about the GPIMM.

See Appendix 1 for details. Contact the author direct if you do not have Web access.

The model defines where a practice is in terms of a maturity level. You may like to think of this as a step on a staircase leading to the level required for the practice to play a full part in the PCG information system:

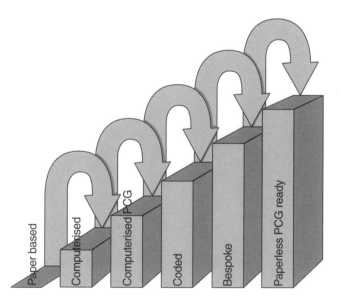

This is why you will find a staircase as the logo of the model. The model is based around five primary maturity levels, with an additional zeroth level for non-computerised practices. The maturity levels are summarised in the table below.

Levels of the GPIMM

Level	Designation	Summary description
0	Paper-based	The practice has no computer system
1	Computerised	The practice has a computer system. It is used only by the practice staff
2	Computerised PHC team	The practice has a computer system. It is used by the practice staff and the PHC team, including the doctors
3	Coded	The system makes limited use of Read Codes
4	Bespoke	The system is tailored to the needs of the practice through agreed coding policies and the use of clinical protocols
5	Paperless	The practice is completely paperless, except where paper records are a legal requirement

The model can help us with two key tasks: identifying where practices are, and identifying what they need to do to make progress. In this chapter we shall deal with how to use the GPIMM to audit where practices are.

The audit is based around a relatively simple questionnaire. This is possible because the model has at its heart a logical model of practice information development. Practices that show different levels of maturity in different areas should consider whether those developments have occurred in a logical fashion. The presence of 'outliers', i.e. higher or lower maturity levels in one area, may be indicative of wasted efforts.

The questionnaire considers five areas to assess maturity:

- *Computerisation* – this is simply a filter to identify those practices that remain paper-based.
- *Personnel usage* – this section looks at the impact of the system on the practice. Systems used only by practice staff are severely limited in their usefulness.
- *Coding* – this section is crucial. It considers not just the extent of coding, but the quality of coding through the extent of policies and consultation underpinning coding practice.
- *System usage* – this section is concerned with the impact that the system has on the working methods of the practice. It measures the extent to which the system works for the practice and not the other way around.
- *Electronic Patient Records* – this section is concerned with the implementation of the Electronic Patient Record. It considers how far the Electronic Patient Record is realised both inside and outside the practice.

The complete questionnaire is given on the next page.

GPIMM maturity level questionnaire

Computerisation

Has the practice got a computerised patient record system installed?

Yes ❏   No   ❏

If No, simply return the questionnaire now.

Personnel usage

Is the system in use within the practice?

Yes ❏   No   ❏

Is the system used by doctors and other members of the primary healthcare team during consultations?

Yes ❏   No   ❏

Coding

Is any information Read Coded by users of the system?

Yes ❏   No   ❏

Has the whole practice adopted standard Read Codes for key clinical areas?

Yes ❏   No   ❏

Are the codes entered subject to a validation procedure?

Yes ❏   No   ❏

Has the practice liaised with other stakeholders, such as other practices within commissioning groups, or the health authority over standard Read Codes?

Yes ❏   No   ❏

Has the practice adopted a policy of 100% coding on patient records?

Yes ❏   No   ❏

GPIMM maturity level questionnaire

System usage

Is the system used to proactively manage repeat prescribing?

Yes ❏   No   ❏

Is the system used to proactively manage acute prescribing?

Yes ❏   No   ❏

Is the system used to proactively manage health promotion?

Yes ❏   No   ❏

Is the system used to implement clinical protocols?

Yes ❏   No   ❏

Is the system used to carry out real-time audits?

Yes ❏   No   ❏

Electronic patient records

Is the system electronically linked to the health authority for transferring information on items of service?

Yes ❏   No   ❏

Is the system fully linked to NHSNet?

Yes ❏   No   ❏

Are paper records only used when legally required?

Yes ❏   No   ❏

The easiest way to implement a GPIMM maturity level is to use the GPIMM-CAPA software tool (General Practice Information Maturity Model-Computer Aided Practice Assessment tool). This software runs under Windows 95 on any PC. The GPIMM-CAPA provides an electronic version of the questionnaire together with an

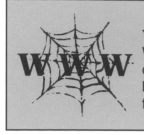
You can download the software tool from the accompanying Web site. See Appendix 1 for details. Contact the author direct if you do not have Web access. Regrettably, there will be a handling charge for sending out the software tool on a floppy disk.

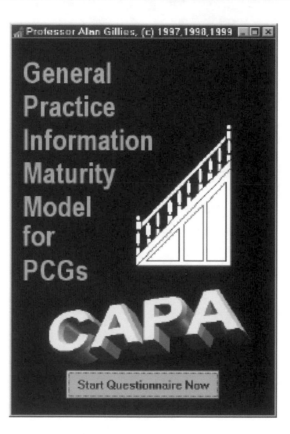

assessment of the current maturity level and further information to be used for practice development in the next chapter.

Using the GPIMM-CAPA tool it is possible to build a profile of the target PCG audience. A simple graph will show at a glance the scale of the problem. Audits of local practices have typically shown the majority of practices at Levels 2 and 3, leaving a lot of work to be done.

A typical practice profile is shown following the CAPA screens.

Fortunately, GPIMM can help us further by identifying and prioritising tasks to be carried out in order to achieve the required level of information management for a successful PCG.

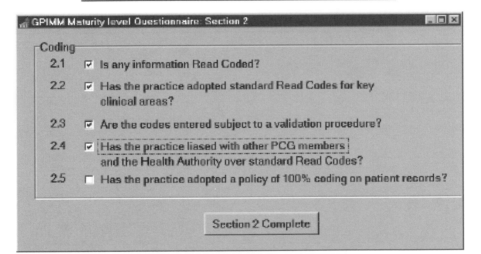

GPIMM Maturity level Questionnaire: Section 0

Computerisation

0.1 ☑ Has the practice got a computerised patient record system?

Section 0 Completed

GPIMM Maturity level Questionnaire: Section 1

Personnel Usage

1.1 ☑ Is the system used by the practice ?

1.2 ☑ Is the system used by the PHC team?

Section 1 Complete

GPIMM Maturity level Questionnaire: Section 2

Coding

2.1 ☑ Is any information Read Coded?

2.2 ☑ Has the practice adopted standard Read Codes for key clinical areas?

2.3 ☑ Are the codes entered subject to a validation procedure?

2.4 ☑ Has the practice liased with other PCG members and the Health Authority over standard Read Codes?

2.5 ☐ Has the practice adopted a policy of 100% coding on patient records?

Section 2 Complete

GPIMM Maturity level Questionnaire: Section 3

System usage

3.1 ☑ Is the system used to proactively manage repeat prescribing?

3.2 ☑ Is the system used to proactively manage acute prescribing?

3.3 ☑ Is the system used to proactively manage health promotion?

3.4 ☑ Is the system used to implement clinical protocols?

3.5 ☑ Is the system used to carry out real time audits?

Section 3 Completed

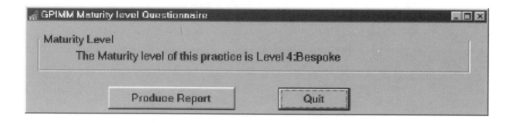

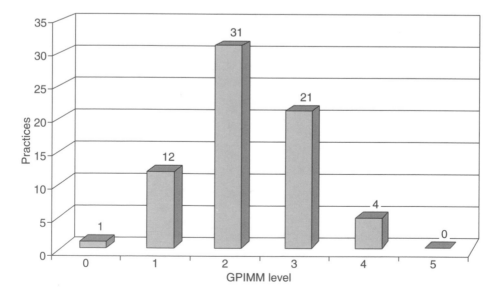

Typical practice profile in terms of GPIMM ca. 1998

Exercise 10

Using the GPIMM-CAPA tool to carry out a GPIMM audit of your practice, what level do you achieve?

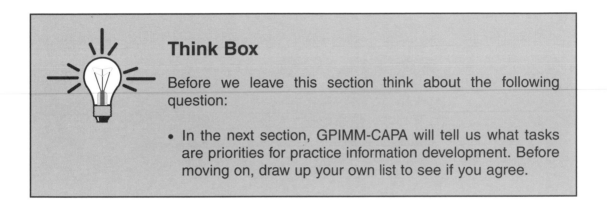

Think Box

Before we leave this section think about the following question:

- In the next section, GPIMM-CAPA will tell us what tasks are priorities for practice information development. Before moving on, draw up your own list to see if you agree.

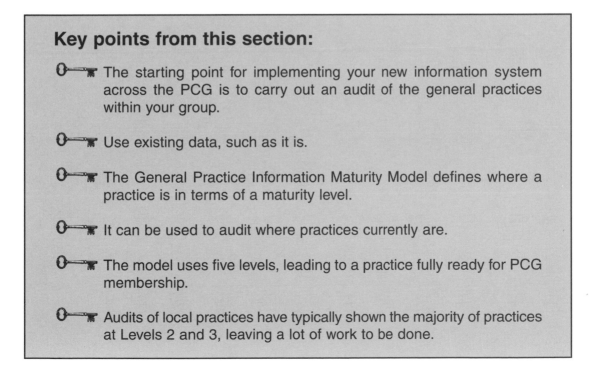

Key points from this section:

⚷ The starting point for implementing your new information system across the PCG is to carry out an audit of the general practices within your group.

⚷ Use existing data, such as it is.

⚷ The General Practice Information Maturity Model defines where a practice is in terms of a maturity level.

⚷ It can be used to audit where practices currently are.

⚷ The model uses five levels, leading to a practice fully ready for PCG membership.

⚷ Audits of local practices have typically shown the majority of practices at Levels 2 and 3, leaving a lot of work to be done.

8

A way forward: information development at the practice level

The GPIMM allows us to define not only the current status of practices, but also a structured practice development path which will provide information strategies to bring each practice up to the required information maturity level to play a full role in the PCG information system.

In this chapter we shall see how this can be achieved. We shall use a typical, if somewhat traditional, practice as a case study to help us.

Case Study Practice 3

Practice 3 is a practice of 12 000 patients with five doctors, based in a suburban New Town area. The practice is based in a purpose built health centre behind a large supermarket. The practice prides itself on the quality of care provided to its patients. It could be summarised as a 'traditional' practice with a stable staff. Their patient list is closed. They have never been a fundholding practice. They are currently using a VAMP computer system. The system is based around the text-based VAMP Medical System, with additional modules for items of service. The practice is linked to the health authority for items of service information.

Case Study Practice 3 *continued*

The current usage of the system is limited. The doctors do not use the system during consultations. Instead, paper notes are used. Information from the paper notes is then entered on to the system at a later date by practice staff. Acute prescriptions are issued manually during consultations.

Similarly, information is extracted from incoming letters by two medical secretaries, who enter key information on to the computer system. None of the information is currently coded.

The practice manager is unhappy with the current situation and would like to move to a system making much greater use of the computer.

The responses to the maturity model questionnaire for this practice are given below.

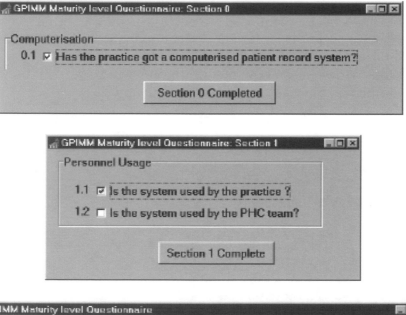

The system automatically logs the practice at Level 1 because of the non-involvement of the doctors. However, we can use the further facilities of the GPIMM-CAPA to make recommendations for practice improvement.

The report produced by entering 'Produce Report' gives the key tasks to be carried out in order to improve information maturity.

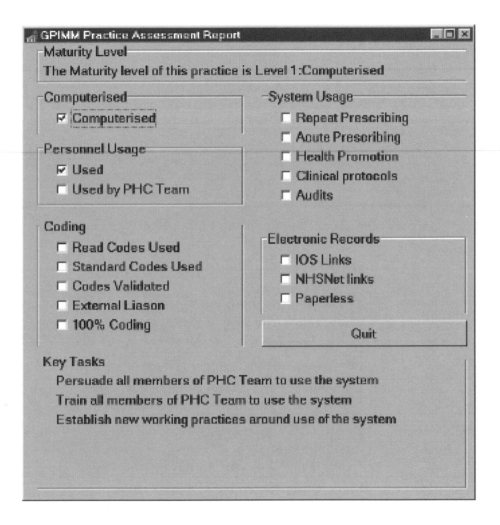

Each level of the GPIMM requires a major change in working practices. It is generally recommended that it should not be attempted to develop practices at a rate of more than one level per year.

✓	**Principle of good practice** Practices need time to change, therefore it is generally recommended that it should not be attempted to develop practices at a rate of more than one level per year.

Therefore, with practices such as this it is necessary to implement a long-term action plan to bring their information to the level required by the PCG. Each year, a GPIMM audit will be needed to check progress against the plan.

The plan for this practice, audited in 1998, is shown in the table below. The report screens from the GPIMM-CAPA screen are shown for the state of the practice in each year.

Action plan to bring practice to required level for PCG

Year	GPIMM level	Tasks to be carried out
1998	1	• Persuade doctors and other PHC workers to use system in consultations • Train PHC team in use of system • Establish new working practices based around use of the system
1999	2	• Persuade all staff to use Read Codes • Train all staff in use of Read Codes • Discuss scope and nature of coding within practice • Liaise with PCG over coding standards • Implement codes within agreed scope
2000	2*	• Implement PCG coding standards with training • Implement practice-defined protocols for diagnosis and prescribing with training • Implement computer-based health promotion policy with training • Implement real-time audits with training
2001	4	• Move all records to electronic form • Agree coding standards with external bodies • Ensure system meets requirements for connection to NHSNet$^{(TB)}$ • Make paper records for legal requirements
2002	5	• Carry out audit to ensure that Level 5 is reached • Implement a culture of continuous monitoring and improvement

*To meet the requirements of Level 3, the practice would have to have implemented computerised repeat prescribing by this year. Once this is achieved, Level 3 will be attained early in 2000.

GPIMM Practice Assessment Report ▬ □ ✕

Maturity Level

The Maturity level of this practice is Level 2:Computerised PHC Team

Computerised
- ☑ Computerised

Personnel Usage
- ☑ Used
- ☑ Used by PHC Team

Coding
- ☐ Read Codes Used
- ☐ Standard Codes Used
- ☐ Codes Validated
- ☐ External Liason
- ☐ 100% Coding

System Usage
- ☐ Repeat Prescribing
- ☐ Acute Prescribing
- ☐ Health Promotion
- ☐ Clinical protocols
- ☐ Audits

Electronic Records
- ☐ IOS Links
- ☐ NHSNet links
- ☐ Paperless

[Quit]

Key Tasks

Persuade all staff to use Read Codes

Train all staff to use Read Codes

Discuss scope and nature of coding within practice

Liase with PCG over coding standards

Implement codes within agreed scope

GPIMM Practice Assessment Report ▬ □ ✕

Maturity Level

The Maturity level of this practice is Level 2:Computerised PHC team

Computerised
- ☑ Computerised

Personnel Usage
- ☑ Used
- ☑ Used by PHC Team

Coding
- ☑ Read Codes Used
- ☑ Standard Codes Used
- ☑ Codes Validated
- ☑ External Liason
- ☐ 100% Coding

System Usage
- ☐ Repeat Prescribing
- ☐ Acute Prescribing
- ☐ Health Promotion
- ☐ Clinical protocols
- ☐ Audits

Electronic Records
- ☑ IOS Links
- ☐ NHSNet links
- ☐ Paperless

[Quit]

Key Tasks

Implement Computerised Repeat Prescribing with training

Implement Computerised Acute Prescribing with training

Implement Computerised Health Promotion with training

Implement Computerised Clinical Protocols with training

Implement real time Clinical Audits with training

Fully code all records

GPIMM Practice Assessment Report

Maturity Level

The Maturity level of this practice is Level 4:Bespoke

Computerised
- ☑ Computerised

Personnel Usage
- ☑ Used
- ☑ Used by PHC Team

Coding
- ☑ Read Codes Used
- ☑ Standard Codes Used
- ☑ Codes Validated
- ☑ External Liason
- ☐ 100% Coding

System Usage
- ☑ Repeat Prescribing
- ☑ Acute Prescribing
- ☑ Health Promotion
- ☑ Clinical protocols
- ☑ Audits

Electronic Records
- ☑ IOS Links
- ☐ NHSNet links
- ☐ Paperless

Quit

Key Tasks

Fully code all records

Ensure system meets with requirements for connection to NHSNet

Computerise remainder, keeping paper records required by law

GPIMM Practice Assessment Report

Maturity Level

The Maturity level of this practice is Level 5:Paperless

Computerised
- ☑ Computerised

Personnel Usage
- ☑ Used
- ☑ Used by PHC Team

Coding
- ☑ Read Codes Used
- ☑ Standard Codes Used
- ☑ Codes Validated
- ☑ External Liason
- ☑ 100% Coding

System Usage
- ☑ Repeat Prescribing
- ☑ Acute Prescribing
- ☑ Health Promotion
- ☑ Clinical protocols
- ☑ Audits

Electronic Records
- ☑ IOS Links
- ☑ NHSNet links
- ☑ Paperless

Quit

Key Tasks

Implement a culture of continuous monitoring and improvement

Exercise 11

 Practice 2 is a practice of 10 000 patients with five doctors. The practice prides itself on being innovative, and was a first wave fund-holding practice. It is based in a suburban area, with new premises developed since the practice became fund holding. The practice is interested in developing health promotion activities and is currently seeking to implement an ischaemic heart disease programme.

They are currently using a VAMP computer system. The system is based around the text-based VAMP Medical System with additional modules for items of service. The practice is linked to the health authority for items of service information.

The system is currently used within consultations by the doctors. Repeat and acute prescriptions are handled by the computer system.

However, none of the information is currently coded. The usage of the system is as a basic recording device with little proactive usage.

Use the GPIMM-CAPA to answer the following:

1 What level of maturity is currently achieved?

2 Draw up an action plan for this practice to reach the required level for participation in the PCG. Enter the action plan in the table below.

Year	GPIMM level	Tasks to be carried out
		• • •
		• • •
		• • •
		• • •
		• • •

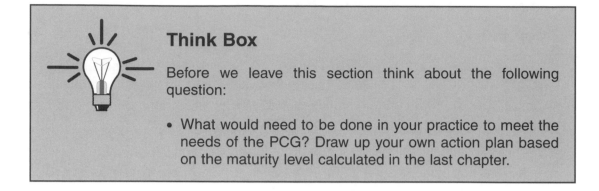

Think Box

Before we leave this section think about the following question:

- What would need to be done in your practice to meet the needs of the PCG? Draw up your own action plan based on the maturity level calculated in the last chapter.

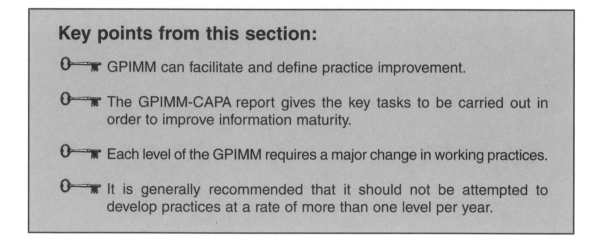

Key points from this section:

⚬━➤ GPIMM can facilitate and define practice improvement.

⚬━➤ The GPIMM-CAPA report gives the key tasks to be carried out in order to improve information maturity.

⚬━➤ Each level of the GPIMM requires a major change in working practices.

⚬━➤ It is generally recommended that it should not be attempted to develop practices at a rate of more than one level per year.

9

So what do we do
at PCG level?

Thus we have seen that the PCG information system is made up of a number of components. The Patient Population Profile in practice can exist as a virtual system. By this we mean that instead of the information existing at PCG level, it exists within the GP systems.

When information is required, instead of the enquirer interrogating a database, they send out a MIQUEST([JB]) query to all the systems and then collate the responses. This could be done in the first instance by disk, but hopefully soon such queries will use the NHSNet to transfer information in both directions. This apparently complex situation provides a number of advantages, which arise from the fact that only one copy of the data exists:

- it prevents duplication of data, which is inefficient
- it prevents potential conflicts between different versions of the data
- it reduces concern over confidentiality
- it encourages partnership between individual practices and the group.

However, this still leaves a number of systems required by the PCG. The author believes that the PCG should hold centrally an age–sex register with basic patient data to facilitate patients moving from practice to practice and other tasks mentioned in earlier chapters. However, this is not accepted by some people.

The PCG will also require a practice database to keep track of practice details. Finally, the PCG should maintain an evidence-based centre to supply evidence guidelines and protocols to the practices for their systems. A schematic of this set-up is shown below.

This means that the main PCG system is a 'front end' or gateway to access information held on other systems. This is what is known as a client server([JB]) system. In this case, the client lives on a PC physically located within the PCG, and two of the systems live on local servers, i.e. servers located with the PCG. The other information lives on servers either in the GP practices, linked hopefully by NHSNet(*JB*), or anywhere in the world connected via the Internet.

This approach does raise a few difficulties. They are summarised opposite.

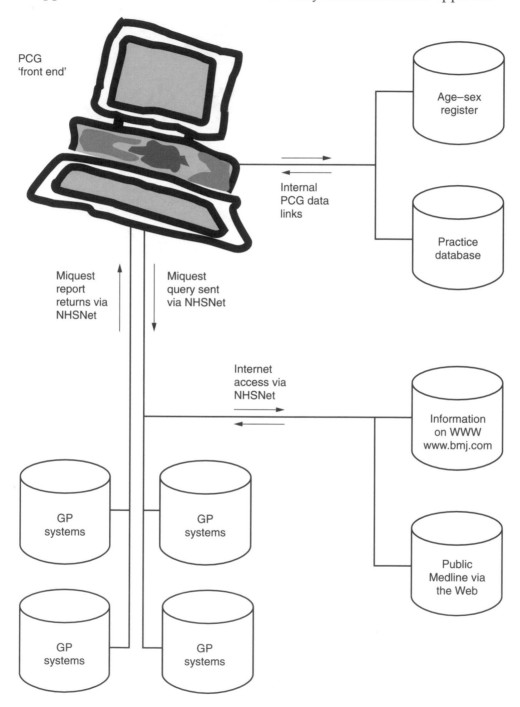

The difficulties of the client server(^{JB}) approach

1 The implementation is technically quite complex.

2 The system is dependent on external links beyond the PCG's direct control.

3 Internet access may open the PCG to external threats such as viruses.

4 NHSNet(^{JB}) may open the PCG to external threats such as viruses.

5 NHSNet(^{JB}) may not be implemented in time.

6 NHSNet(^{JB}) may not work!

These may be summarised under two headings:

- technical complexity
- dependency upon the NHSNet(^{JB}).

Although the technical complexity is quite high, client server(^{JB}) systems are the norm in most systems of any size. The most common type of client server system occurs when a home PC user logs on to the Internet. This turns the humble PC into a client server(^{JB}) system of really ferocious complexity. Fortunately, most of this is hidden behind the innocent Internet Explorer screen. This is exactly how the PCG system should be, with the complexity all hidden away from the user.

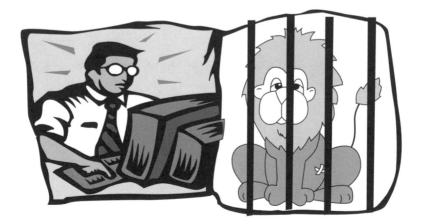

Within a client server environment something really ferocious may lurk behind the screen, but should be hidden from the user!

The second issue is the NHSNet(^{JB}). There is a political imperative to ensure that every GP practice is physically connected to the NHSNet(^{JB}) during 1999. Therefore we may assume that this will happen, maybe even by the time you read this.

However, getting connected to the NHSNet(^{JB}) is somewhat more complex than plugging in to a wall socket. There are significant issues surrounding control of access, security and confidentiality.

But there is more. The really big problem is sending messages across the NHSNet(^{JB}) from one incompatible system to another. Therefore, the mode of use of the NHSNet(^{JB}) is likely to be limited for some time to come. Therefore, in this book we have limited our use to reflect this.

For the foreseeable future, the NHSNet(^{JB}) is likely to be limited to the following functions:

Functions of NHSNet(^{JB}) likely to be available 'soon'

1 Electronic mail for the transmission of plain text messages.

2 Electronic mail for the transmission of binary computer files as attachments to messages. This will facilitate the exchange of MIQUEST(^{JB}) queries and reports, essential to our implementation of a PCG information system. Also the sending of guidelines and protocols to practices for use with their proprietary systems.

3 Access to the Internet and to other on-line services, giving access to Department of Health documents, Medline, electronic journals, such as the *BMJ*, and evidence-based sites such as the Cochrane databases and Bandolier.

Using the NHSNet(^{JB}) in this way should ensure that the level of service described is available in the near future. Failing this, these functions can be duplicated by a box of floppy disks and access to an independent Internet connection.

Exercise 12

Find out what information systems are currently run by the health authority to cover the functions that will be run by the PCG, once it reaches maturity. Remember that such systems may be paper-based as well as computerised. Use the table below to identify the systems, using the format column to identify whether the system is currently paper-based or computerised.

Health authority system	Format	Proposed PCG system

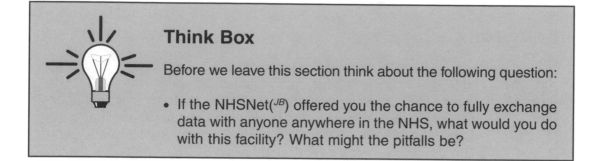

Think Box

Before we leave this section think about the following question:

- If the NHSNet(^{JB}) offered you the chance to fully exchange data with anyone anywhere in the NHS, what would you do with this facility? What might the pitfalls be?

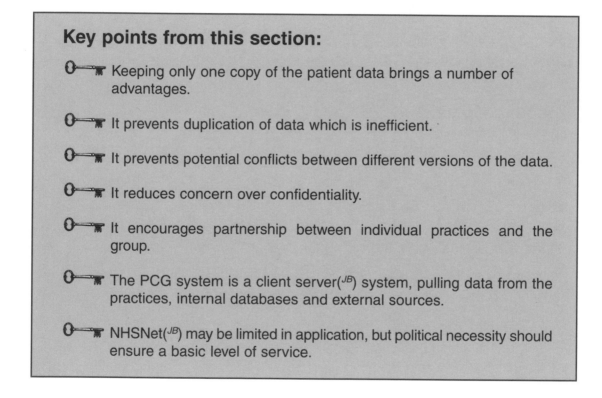

Key points from this section:

🔑 Keeping only one copy of the patient data brings a number of advantages.

🔑 It prevents duplication of data which is inefficient.

🔑 It prevents potential conflicts between different versions of the data.

🔑 It reduces concern over confidentiality.

🔑 It encourages partnership between individual practices and the group.

🔑 The PCG system is a client server(^{JB}) system, pulling data from the practices, internal databases and external sources.

🔑 NHSNet(^{JB}) may be limited in application, but political necessity should ensure a basic level of service.

10

How to avoid buying
a white elephant

Computer purchases are expensive, and they can be tricky. However, the NHS does have procedures for buying things and these can be applied to computers as well as to anything else. The basis for this is the procurement process, which can be based on the NHS procurement procedure, known as POISE. The information strategy document either for an individual practice or the PCG will form part of the business case. The business case is a key stage in the POISE process shown below.

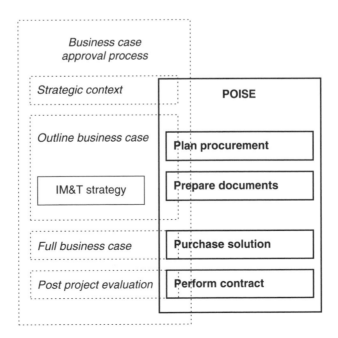

The POISE methodology helps you go about things in a structured and systematic way. It should help you make sure that you have done all the things you should. But remember the importance of people as well as process.

> ## ✓ Principle of good practice
>
> Involve all the people – and get good advice from people you can trust.

We shall look at an example of the information strategy of a real business case, prepared by the author to help two practices trying to purchase similar systems to enable them to share data.

> ## 💼 Case Study 4 Practices A and B
>
> As part of the outline business case, this document will take the procurement procedure as far as the preparation of a shortlist of two systems.
>
> The next section will describe the planning for procurement and will include those elements of the POISE PID not specified elsewhere in the business case.
>
> ### Planning for procurement
> The scope of the procurement covered by this document is the procurement of two patient record systems, one for each of the organisations. The projected budget for each system is approximately £70 000, but this does not include training requirements additional to the initial training supplied as part of the purchase.
>
> The GP system marketplace, from which the system must be acquired, is dominated by a small number of suppliers. In a 1995 survey of systems in Lancashire, shown below, the author found that five suppliers provided systems for 67% of the practices. Data supplied by the NHSE (NorthWest) for the whole North West region in 1997 shows that EMIS has gained market share.

Case Study 4 Practices A and B *continued*

These five suppliers were contacted along with several others to provide information for the procurement process. The suppliers were asked to supply technical and financial information, information about compliance to RFA4 (Rules for Accreditation)([JB]), the nearest thing available to an agreed national specification for a GP system, and finally specific information with regard to Year 2000 compliance to prevent problems arising in this area. The actual questionnaire used is appended to this report.

In addition to this basic information, the views of key stakeholders were taken into account:

- From Practice A:

'We do not want another Supplier 1 system because we are not satisfied with the level of support offered by the company.'

'Usability is of prime importance.'

- From the Acute Trust:

'We support links with Supplier 1, Supplier 2 and Supplier 3 systems.'

In addition, to maximise the benefit derived from the main system, the patient record system should be complemented with office software to facilitate word processing, analysis and presentation of data extracted from the main system. This will involve no further hardware investment but will cost an additional £300 per workstation in software costs.

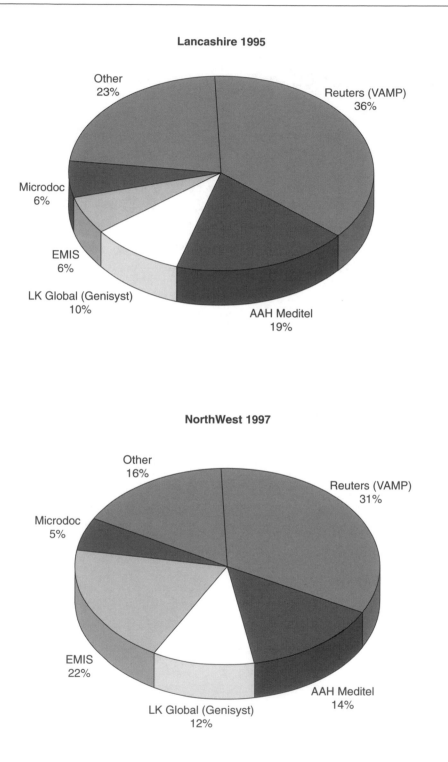

Lancashire 1995

Other
23%

Reuters (VAMP)
36%

Microdoc
6%

EMIS
6%

LK Global (Genisyst)
10%

AAH Meditel
19%

NorthWest 1997

Other
16%

Microdoc
5%

Reuters (VAMP)
31%

EMIS
22%

LK Global (Genisyst)
12%

AAH Meditel
14%

Results of planning process

Table 10.1 The results of the questionnaire survey from the main suppliers

	System 1	System 2	System 3	System 4	System 5
Operating system	W3.11/NT	NT/W95	Unix	W95/DOS	Unix/W95
Server CPU	P200	P200	P200	P200	P200
Server RAM	64Mb	64Mb	32Mb	32Mb	32Mb
Server disk	4Gb	2Gb	5Gb	5Gb	4Gb
Client CPU	P200	P166	P166	P166	P166
Client RAM	32Mb	16Mb	16Mb	16Mb	16Mb
Client disk	1.6Gb	1.2Gb	2Gb	2Gb	2Gb
Example price[2]	£50K	£35K	£40K	£28K	£50K
RFA4 1.1	✓	✓	✓	✓	✓
RFA4 1.2	✓	✓	✓	✓	✓
RFA4 1.3	✓	✓	✓	✓	✓
RFA4 2.1	✓	✓	✓	✓	✓
RFA4 2.2	✓	✓	✓	✓	✓
RFA4 3.1	✓	✓	✓	✓	✓
RFA4 3.2	✓	✓	✓	✓	✓
RFA4 3.3	✓	✓	✓	✓	✓
RFA4 3.4	✓	✓	✓	✓	✓
RFA4 3.5	✓	✓	✓	✓	✓
RFA4 3.6	✓	✓	✓	✓	✓
RFA4 3.7	✓	✓	✓	✓	✓
RFA4 4.1	✓	✓	✓	✓	✓
RFA4 4.2	✓	✓	✓	✓	✓
RFA4 4.3	✓	✓	✓	✓	✓
RFA4 4.4	✓	✓	✓	✓	✓
RFA4 4.5	✓	✓	✓	✓	✓
RFA4 4.6	✓	✓	✓	✓	✓
RFA4 5.1	✓	✓	✓	✓	✓
RFA4 5.2	✓	✓	✓	✓	✓
RFA4 5.3	✓	✓	✓	✓	✓
RFA4 5.4	✓	✓	✓	✓	✓
RFA4 5.5	✓	✓	✓	✓	✓
RFA4 6.1	✓	✓	✓	✓	✓
RFA4 6.2	✓	✓	✓	✓	✓
RFA4 6.3	✓	✓	✓	✓	✓
RFA4 6.4	✓	✓	✓	✓	✓
RFA4 6.5	✓	✓	✓	✓	✓
External acc.	Nil	RFA1	RFA2	RFA1	(RFA4)[3]
Date storage	?[4]	✓	✓	✓	✓
Date input	?[4]	✓	✓	✓	✓
29 Feb 2000	?[4]	✓	✓	✓	✓
Rollover	?[4]	Auto	Auto	Auto	Auto
Backwards	?[4]	N/A	✓	✓	N/A
Testing[5]	?[4]	Int.	Int.	Ext.	RFA4

[1] The remaining three suppliers contacted did not respond.
[2] Example comparative price quoted for ten PC systems per site.
[3] Due November 1997.
[4] The supplier response gave no guarantees of compliance.
[5] Int. = internal testing, Ext. = independent testing, RFA4 = independent RFA4 test.

Table 10.2 shows data supplied by Exeter systems, responsible for the accreditation of GP systems, giving a more complete picture of accreditation status of the major systems. Please note that this data was accurate at the time of the work (autumn 1997).

The survey shows that all the major suppliers believe that their systems do comply with the RFA4 regulations. However, Table 10.2 shows that there is currently no external validation of this. In view of this it is recommended that any contract includes a clause which makes RFA4 compliance a legally binding requirement. Of the systems included in Table 10.1, only the Supplier 5 system offers a date for RFA4 level accreditation, within one month of this report.

Table 10.2 Accreditation status supplied by Exeter systems							
Feature	GP systems						
	Supplier 1		Supplier 2		Supplier 3	Supplier 4	Supplier 5
Accreditation	System 1a	System 1b	System 2a	System 2b	System 3	System 4	System 5
Requirements for accreditation							
RFA4	✗	✗	✗	✗	✗	✗	✗
RFA3	✗	✗	✗	✗	✗	✓	✗
RFA2	✗	✗	✗	✓	✗	✓	✗
RFA1	✓	✓	✓	✓	✓	✓	✓
HA/GP Links registration							
Phase 1 conformance	✓	✓	✓	✓	✓	✓	✓
Phase 1 completed pilot	✓	✓	✓	✓	✓	✓	✓
Phase 2 conformance	✗	✗	✗	✗	✗	✓	✓
Phase 2 completed pilot	✗	✗	✗	✗	✗	✗	✗
HA/GP links items of service							
Conformance	✓	✓	✓	✓	✓	✓	✓
Completed pilot	✓	✓	✓	✓	✓	✓	✓
X400							
Conformance	✗	✗	✗	✗	✗	✓	✗
Completed pilot	✗	✗	✗		✗	✗	✗
Provider links							
Pathology reports	✗	✗	✗	✗	✗	✗	✗
Radiology reports	✗	✗	✗	✗	✗	✗	✗
Discharge notifications	✗	✗	✗	✗	✗	✗	✗
PNL	✗	✗	✗	✗	✗	✗	✗

If we consider each system in terms of the criteria then the results are shown Table 10.3.

Table 10.3					
	System 1	System 2	System 3	System 4	System 5
Within budget	✓	✓	✓	✓	✓
RFA4	✓	✓	✓	✓	✓
Externally verified	✗	✗	✗	✗	✓
Year 2000	✗	✓	✓	✓	✓
Externally verified	✗	✗	✗	✗	✗
User friendly[1]	✓	✓	✓	✗	✓
Not supplier 1[2]	✗	✓	✓	✓	✓
Hospital supported	✓	✓	✓	✗	✗

[1] User friendly is simplistically defined as a graphical interface and a second-generation system
[2] Practice A will not consider Supplier 1.

From this summary analysis, System 1 is ruled out because Practice A will not countenance another system from that supplier. Their Year 2000 compliance is also less satisfactory from the supplier survey. Similarly, Supplier 5 does not fit Practice A's requirements for a user-friendly system. Since hospital links form a key part of the IM&T(*JB*) strategy, the criterion of hospital support favours System 2 and System 3. Of the other two, System 5 is worthy of note because of its RFA4 accreditation. However, if claims made in the procurement survey are made explicitly legally binding in the contract, then this advantage is diminished.

Final stages of procurement

The final stages of procurement, taken from the POISE procedure, are shortlist and negotiation.

From the process outlined above, we have arrived at a shortlist of two suppliers. From this point, each supplier should be invited to submit a detailed specification and provide demonstrations for the organisations. The final decision should be made on the following criteria:

- match to detailed information needs
- match to detailed usability requirements, including, for example, can the doctors use it during a consultation?
- support and training package
- cost.

Recommendations

- It is recommended that Systems 2 and 3 should form a shortlist from which the final system choice is made.
- It is further recommended that the suppliers should be asked to sign an undertaking that information submitted during procurement concerning RFA4 compliance is legally binding.
- It is recommended that each workstation also includes a standard suite of office software to maximise the benefits from the main system.

This kind of structured analysis process can be very helpful. However, it is also important that the views of all stakeholders are taken into account. For example, in the above case study, the practice manager had the following to say about their existing supplier and system (Supplier 1).

Staff and practice manager problems
with existing system

- Very limited initial training (4 hours).
- Difficulty in constructing search templates to extract required information.
- Problems with communication links in the IOS Module.
- Lack of responsibility for above problems between system supplier, communications supplier and health authority.
- Very poor support and helpline.
- High turnover of contact staff.
- Difficult to reconcile information on system with information supplied by health authority.
- Poor user interface design leading to complex tasks on cluttered screens.
- Doctors discouraged from using the system because of the time taken to input data arising from user's interface design.
- System designed to recognise words from initial letters ineffective.
- Call/recall system does not take account of patient coming early for appointment.
- Staff were unaware of existing functions due to lack of training, support and poor usability of system.

Even if Supplier 1's newer system was the best option, the legacy of a bad experience particularly with support and training is likely to make implementation very difficult. This kind of feeling strongly expressed is ignored at great peril.

Exercise 13

The table below is a rather simpler version of the table used in the case study.

The leading new GP systems in terms of market share are Vamp Vision, Meditel System 6000 and EMIS.

By contacting suppliers and by referring to the RFA accreditation Web site at http://www.fhs.org.uk/pages/services/accred/list.htm (which is accessible from the Web pages associated with this book) evaluate these systems using the table. You may like to supplement this by interviewing practice members to establish their views.

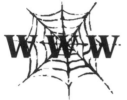

To complete this exercise fully does require access to the World Wide Web. However, gathering information from suppliers is possible without WWW access, as is the staff interview part of the exercise.

	System 1	System 2	System 3
Operating system			
Server CPU			
Server RAM			
Server disk			
Client CPU			
Client RAM			
Client disk			
Example price			
Within budget			
RFA4 claimed			
Externally verified			
RFA3 accreditation			
RFA2 accreditation			
Year 2000 claimed			
Externally verified			
Graphical user interface			
Hospital supported			

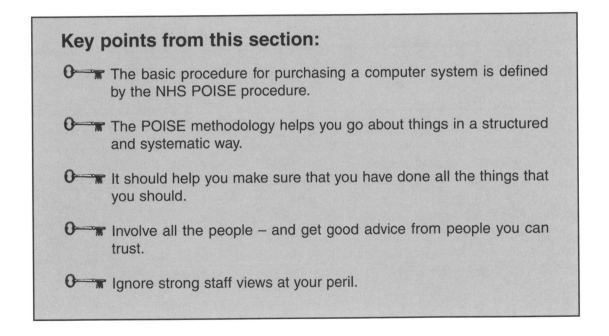

Think Box

Before we leave this section think about the following question:

- If you were to acquire one of the new shiny systems evaluated above, what clinical benefits might accrue? Would it help your practice play a more effective role in the PCG?

Key points from this section:

The basic procedure for purchasing a computer system is defined by the NHS POISE procedure.

The POISE methodology helps you go about things in a structured and systematic way.

It should help you make sure that you have done all the things that you should.

Involve all the people – and get good advice from people you can trust.

Ignore strong staff views at your peril.

11

Keeping the PCG
out of jail

It is an oft-heard cry that 'you can't do that – it's against the Data Protection Act'. However, there is much ignorance about the Act, and it certainly can be used as a smokescreen for not providing access to information.

In principle there are two types of things that you can't do. The first is things that the law says you can't do. The second are things that you could do legitimately if you identified them on your data protection entry with the Data Protection Registrar.

The extent of the problem is best illustrated by a local survey carried out by a Family Health Service Authority IT manager in 1992. It revealed that over 90% of general practices in his area had inadequacies in their data protection entry, some of which were serious enough to lead to prosecution and possible unlimited fines.

The UK Data Protection Act was enacted in 1984. It placed a number of requirements on any organisation holding personal information on computer.

Principles of good practice

Since 1984, practices and health authorities have been required to:

1 identify what information is held on computer

2 identify the purpose for which it is used

3 identify a Data Protection Officer responsible for this area

4 send this information to the Data Protection Registrar as an entry for the Data Protection Register

5 keep this entry up to date.

It is the final requirement that has generally been lacking in most general practices. As computer usage has grown since the mid-1980s, so the data protection entries have often failed to keep up.

However, data protection should be a natural part of professional practice as it is simply part of patient confidentiality.

The 1984 Act was updated in 1998 to bring the Act into line with EU Data Protection Directive (95/46/EC). Much of this was already covered in the earlier Act. The biggest change was to remove the distinction between paper- and computer-based data.

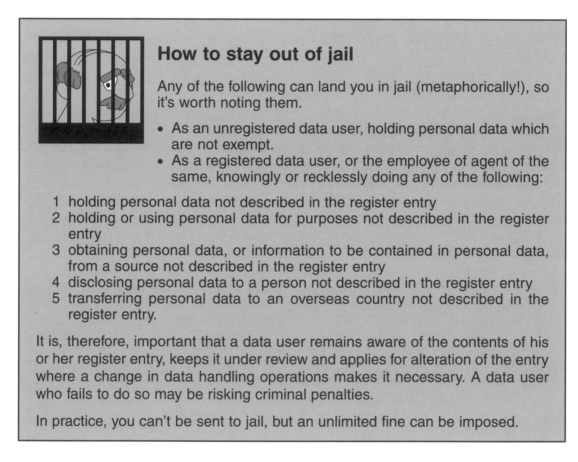

How to stay out of jail

Any of the following can land you in jail (metaphorically!), so it's worth noting them.

- As an unregistered data user, holding personal data which are not exempt.
- As a registered data user, or the employee of agent of the same, knowingly or recklessly doing any of the following:

1 holding personal data not described in the register entry
2 holding or using personal data for purposes not described in the register entry
3 obtaining personal data, or information to be contained in personal data, from a source not described in the register entry
4 disclosing personal data to a person not described in the register entry
5 transferring personal data to an overseas country not described in the register entry.

It is, therefore, important that a data user remains aware of the contents of his or her register entry, keeps it under review and applies for alteration of the entry where a change in data handling operations makes it necessary. A data user who fails to do so may be risking criminal penalties.

In practice, you can't be sent to jail, but an unlimited fine can be imposed.

The practical implication is that every practice in the PCG and the PCG itself must maintain an accurate and up-to-date data protection entry on the Data Protection Register. However, in practice, PCGs operating at Levels 1 and 2 remain part of the health authority and may be covered by their data protection entry. Please check!

To establish a new entry for a new practice or PCG, telephone the Data Protection Registrar's office. The Registrar will take basic details and send out an application form. (It's a DPR1 for people who love Read Codes and other similar things!)

This comes in three parts, Part A, Part B and no, not part C, but the declaration. Part A contains basic contact information, whether the practice is a data user only or a computer bureau (the answer to this question is left as an exercise for the reader!) and the period of registration (1, 2, or 3 years).

You may need more than one Part B. You must fill in a Part B for every purpose for which you hold personal data. Examples of relevant purposes might include the provision of healthcare, clinical research, employee management.

Part B comes in 4 sections:

- B1 is a description of the purpose for which the data is to be held or used
- B2 is a description of the data itself
- B3 is a description of the sources from which the data will be obtained
- B4 is a description of the overseas countries to which the data may be transferred!

The declaration is simply to be signed and the form returned to the Data Protection Registrar's office. The data protection entry is summarised schematically below.

Form DPR1		
Section A Basic contact details for registered data user	**Section B1** Purpose for which the data are to be held or used	
	Section B2 Data to be held or used	
	Section B3 Sources from which the data are to be gathered	
	Section B4 Overseas countries to which the data may be transferred!	
Declaration:	Signed: *Data User*	Dated: *01/01/2000*

In practice, you are more likely to be modifying an existing entry. For this you need a different form (the DPR2, in a triumph of sequential logic!) which may be used to modify any of the above sections.

Exercise 14

 Investigate the data protection entry for your practice. Fill in the schematic entry below from your findings:

Form DPR1	
Section A	**Section B1**
	Section B2
	Section B3
	Section B4
Declaration: Signed: Dated:	

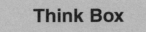

Think Box

Before we leave this section think about the following question:

- What are the implications for your data protection entry of being part of a PCG? You may like to consider sections B1 to B3 in turn.

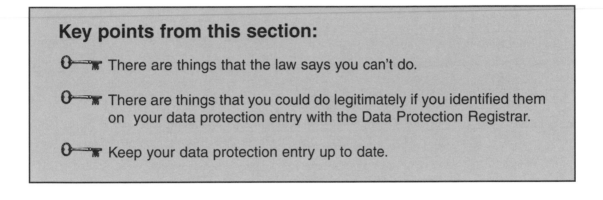

Key points from this section:

There are things that the law says you can't do.

There are things that you could do legitimately if you identified them on your data protection entry with the Data Protection Registrar.

Keep your data protection entry up to date.

12

Just when you thought it
was all under control

The final fly in the ointment (well, at least the last that I'm going to deal with in this book) is the need for PCGs to work with other non-NHS agencies. Under the stated objectives is the following:

> better integrate primary and community health services and work more closely with social services on both planning and delivery. Services such as child health or rehabilitation where responsibilities have been split within the health service and where liaison with Local Authorities is often poor, will particularly benefit

> (*The New NHS* White Paper, 1997)

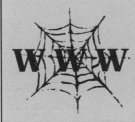 This comes from *The New NHS* White Paper of 1997. The full document is available on the World Wide Web and may be accessed via the Web site associated with this book. See Appendix 1 for details. A full paper reference is given in Appendix 2.

This will require the integration, or at least the exchange, of information between the PCG and social services. This is not really a problem from a technical perspective. Our client server(^{IB}) system is flexible enough to add another server, this time physically located within social services. The modified schematic is shown below.

The more significant problems are organisational and cultural. By now, if you're still reading the book, you'll have gathered that it is held to be self-evident within this book that *information* is king, *not* information *technology*.

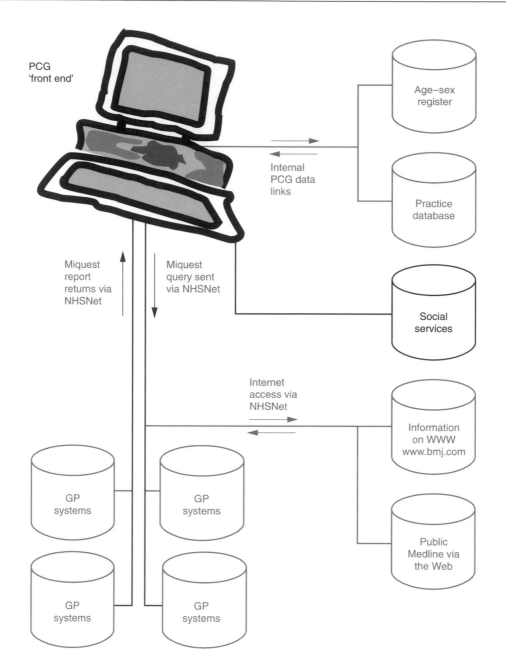

PCG
'front end'

Age–sex register

Internal PCG data links

Practice database

Miquest report returns via NHSNet

Miquest query sent via NHSNet

Social services

Internet access via NHSNet

Information on WWW www.bmj.com

GP systems

GP systems

Public Medline via the Web

GP systems

GP systems

Studies by the author in the areas of mental health and childcare have revealed fundamental differences between the way that social care and healthcare organisations operate and the way they view information. Any PCG wishing to improve collaborative working with their local social care agencies must recognise these differences and take steps to negotiate compromises between agencies to take account of them.

What healthcare agencies do	What social care agencies do
Coding schemes	
Read Codes, probably version 2	Incompatible local authority codes
Fundamental information entities	
Patient-based health records	Family unit records
Attitudes to information collecting	
More information is better	Only information leading to specific actions should be collected
Attitudes to confidentiality	
Information may be shared amongst primary care team	Information should be tightly restricted
Information rarely stigmatises	Information can stigmatise

We shall consider the implications of each in turn.

Coding

The coding of information is crucial to its effective management by computer-based information systems. Two key issues emerge in relation to coding in the inter-agency context. The first is the choice of coding systems. Within primary healthcare, the coding system now reaching universal acceptance is Read Codes. There appears to be little alternative to the use of Read Codes as the basis of recording health data for inter-agency working. This will provide potential integration with the primary care electronic patient record. However, it is not likely that Read Codes will be accepted readily by other agencies. Further it is unclear that Read Codes can provide a universal coding standard for the information required to be contained within inter-agency working. One of the most helpful tools to assist joint working would be a mapping to convert key social care codes into Read Codes.

Experience from the CHDGP data collection project suggests that the other major issue is the quality and consistency of coding. This is simply an extension of the issues discussed for intra-PCG working.

Fundamental information entities

Within any system, a crucial definition is the basic entity around which the system is built. Within an entity relationship model, the model is defined in terms of entities and the relationships between them. In most systems, either one entity is central or perhaps a system may be built around a relationship between two key entities, e.g. library systems are defined by the relationship between borrowers and books (or other items). Clinical systems tend to be patient-focused; crucially information is linked to a single individual. This maps well on to the clinician–patient relationship and mode of working.

In social care, particularly in the context of children, the basic relationship is often with a family as a collective unit. This raises a number of issues. In data modelling terms, the issue becomes whether to model the family as a subentity of individual children or vice versa. As one family may have many children, it is more logical to use the family as the basic entity. However, this is then in conflict with the clinical perspective where information relates to an individual. The PCG client will need to identify data held by social services about families with the specific individual children belonging to that family unit.

Attitudes to information collecting

In the healthcare sector generally, there is a view that the more information collected the better, since this provides a richer picture of the health of the patient. Particularly in primary care, a wide range of factors may influence the health of the patient, and the immediate symptoms and stated reason for consulting the doctor may not be the most significant factors.

This has sometimes had a negative influence on GP systems which have tended to become 'sinks' for information with little thought as to when the information may be retrieved and in what form.

By contrast, social workers tend to be much more minimalist in their information collection, preferring to emphasise that only relevant and targeted information, which is linked to specific courses of action, is collected. This has been explained in terms of the fear of litigation. This derives from cases where, following a failure of care, it can be shown that information was available and not acted upon.

The PCG may find the social care agencies less than grateful for a drip feed of inconclusive pieces of information relating to problems with children at risk or mental health patients housed in the community.

System usage must therefore be defined within agreed protocols, where it is clearly defined at what point action is required on the part of an individual professional or manager. However, it is recognised that even this may not be enough to 'sell' the system if a culture of fear exists.

Attitudes to confidentiality

Although health data is appropriately regarded as 'sensitive', the information in most child health records is not as sensitive as that relating to children being classified as 'at risk'. Much child health data is routine, e.g. recording the occurrence of childhood diseases. These data carry no stigma.

The very act of recording that a child may be at risk is extremely sensitive and changes the nature and context of all information regarding that child. For example, a child arriving at A&E with a fracture, with no history or label attached, is likely to receive only sympathetic treatment. The knowledge that this child has been deemed to be 'at risk' changes the nature of the information from a simple clinical diagnosis with consequences limited to treatment of the injury to potentially crucial evidence of significant abuse.

Thus, professional and parental attitudes to the information are likely to be fundamentally different. There is no significant need for excessive confidentiality over an incident such as a fracture arising from a genuine accident, unless there is a belief that the injury is caused by deliberate harm.

PCGs are increasingly likely to function as teams of practices themselves operating as teams. Thus, increasingly, healthcare is managed as a team activity. In most circumstances, it is professionally acceptable for all members of a team involved in the healthcare of a patient to have access to all relevant information.

However, the number of professionals involved in the process of care for a child deemed to be at risk may be considerable and the degree of their involvement may vary significantly. Therefore, it is appropriate to define a hierarchical model of access to sensitive information on a 'need to know' basis. For example, teachers and police officers may be involved in the process but need to have only partial knowledge. Within a school, there may be further differentiation between teachers designated to deal with child abuse cases, teachers with direct pastoral responsibility, such as form or year tutors, and class teachers.

This level of access may also apply to data input. In considering protocols, such as those suggested above, it may be appropriate to set different thresholds for action based on the specific training and experience of the person making the entry on the system. An alternative may be to restrict access to any information to facilitate human scrutiny by experienced and trained personnel of all reports made to the system.

Agreement over these issues, or indeed a lack of it, is likely to have a much greater impact upon the working of the PCG in inter-agency working than technical limitations.

Exercise 15

A school nurse reports a child as showing unusual bruising and being unusually quiet. What needs to be done and who holds relevant information? Use the table below to consider this problem in terms of:

- Who should act?
- What should they do?
- What information do they need to act?
- Who holds that information?

Who should act?	What should they do?	What information do they need?	Who holds that information?

Think Box

Before we leave this section think about the following question:

- In the scenario considered in Exercise 12, how might an effective PCG information system improve things? What are the key steps required to implement such a system?

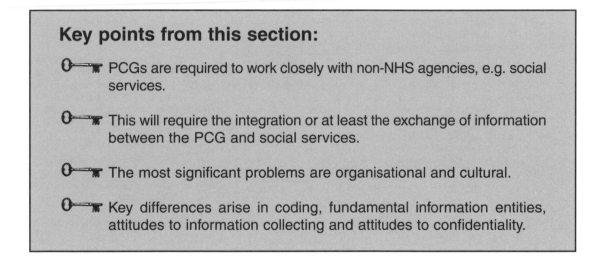

Key points from this section:

⚬━🗝 PCGs are required to work closely with non-NHS agencies, e.g. social services.

⚬━🗝 This will require the integration or at least the exchange of information between the PCG and social services.

⚬━🗝 The most significant problems are organisational and cultural.

⚬━🗝 Key differences arise in coding, fundamental information entities, attitudes to information collecting and attitudes to confidentiality.

13

Some things that might just make it all worthwhile

Why bother? It's a bit late to ask that, you may say. Inevitably, this book has focused on the pitfalls. Hopefully, you've found some solutions, too. But the real measure of success will be if in five years' time, PCGs have effective information systems and these are delivering better care as a consequence.

General practice and PCGs have the opportunity to deliver the most powerful health information database ever seen, probably anywhere in the world as, strange as it may seem, in clinical information, UK general practice probably leads the world. Can it happen? Yes it can. And the evidence lies in Scotland. It's time for another of those fairy stories.

Once upon a time ... (well in 1993, actually)

... a mad professor, to whom nobody was going to listen, went to Disneyland in Florida. There, in sight of an enchanted castle, he displayed a poster at an obscure American computing conference. The poster said:

> The computerisation of doctors' surgeries within the National Health Service (NHS) in the UK has proceeded along different lines in England and Wales in comparison with Scotland.
>
> In England and Wales the process has been driven by the private sector, with a range of commercial companies competing to sell their proprietary products to general practitioners (GPs). The dominant feature in this approach has been competition.

In Scotland, the process has been driven by the regional health bodies, who have provided free software for practices, thus ensuring that over 90% of those practices who are computerised use the same (GPASS) system.

The English computerisation has been dominated by a competitive free market ethos, leading to:

- competition between suppliers

- higher costs to practices

- more advanced technology

- data incompatibility

- poor training.

The Scottish experience has been characterised by centralised provision, leading to:

- single system provided free

- low cost to practices

- less advanced technology

- compatible data: good training.

The mad professor was noticed and everyone said how sensible the Scottish system was and how useful it would be if every GP system in England could talk to each other.

So they all went away and designed systems that could do this and the mad professor lived happily ever after.

However, this being real life and 1993, in practice everyone stayed wedded to their ideological purity and kept on building systems which served the isolationist ideology of fundholding very well. The professor eventually got his work published in a rather good academic information systems journal which was safely off the reading list of any GP or indeed NHS IM&T([JB]) personnel.

Meanwhile, back in Scotland, isolationism meant rejecting the competitive Sassenach (roughly translated, this means English) policies such as fundholding. In Scotland, in excess of 80% of practices use a common piece of software known as GPASS. In 1996, studies showed that the quality of data available from aggregating GPASS data was at least as good as that in hospital systems.

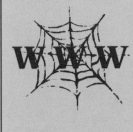 This study was published in the *British Journal of General Practice* by Whitelaw FG *et al.* in 1996 with the title 'Completeness and accuracy of morbidity and repeat prescribing records held on general practice computers in Scotland'. The Abstract may be accessed via public access Medline accessed through the Web pages associated with this book.

You may also wish to refer to the GPASS Data Evaluation Project Web site accessible via the same route.

At the University of Aberdeen, work based on aggregated data has been carrying on. Data are collated in two ways. An electronic questionnaire is used to gather data from 460 practices covering in excess of two million patients. More complete data are gathered from a Continuous Morbidity Reporting System, currently being piloted with 52 practices, with plans to expand across Scotland. The areas of coverage provided by this system are given below.

Data type	Electronic questionnaire (EQ)	Continuous Morbidity Reporting (CMR)
Patient-based data	✓	✓
Practice-based data	✓	✓
Workload – doctors		✓
Workload – nurses		Pilot study
Numeric summary	✓	✓
Numeric details		✓
Morbidity	Major diseases	All diseases
Symptoms		✓
Diagnoses	Major diseases	All diseases
Encounters		✓
Episodes of care		✓
Resource-related groups	Major diseases	All diseases
Repeat prescribing	✓	✓
Acute prescribing	Partial	Partial
Health promotion	✓	✓
Chronic disease management	Major diseases	All diseases
Immunisation	✓	✓
Cervical cytology	✓	✓
Screening	✓	✓
Administration	✓	✓

The data analysis facilitated by the continuous morbidity reporting is more extensive than the questionnaire.

Data type	Electronic questionnaire (EQ)	Continuous Morbidity Reporting (CMR)
Age–sex profiles	✓	✓
Workload encounter data		✓
Incidence/prevalence		✓
Acute, chronic long-term disease		✓
Post code/geographic distribution	✓	✓
Post code/deprivation	✓	✓
Frequency profiles	Major diseases	✓
Doctor/patient behaviour		✓
Time studies		✓
Seasonality		✓
Epidemics		✓
Community data		✓
Prescribing data	✓	✓
Referral data	Partial	Partial
Use of resources		✓
Read Codes by symptoms		✓
Read Codes by individual	Major diseases	✓
Read Codes by group	Major diseases	✓
Read Codes by hierarchy	Major diseases	✓
Read Codes by population	Major diseases	✓
Read Codes by disease	Major diseases	✓
Read Codes by range of morbidity	Incomplete	✓
Read Codes by morbidity associations		✓

Isn't it nice to know that in this information age, GPs from five practices in Orkney and their 11 000 patients have access to better data than colleagues in London? And all because they recognised the value of talking to each other at a much earlier stage.

Even the simpler electronic questionnaire gives information, allowing analysis by postcode. It is this kind of information that is essential to effective local commissioning, which is the core activity of PCGs.

The Scottish experience demonstrates that it is possible to produce information that will support effective local healthcare for a local population.

As a final note, I shall finish with ten things that PCGs could do with effective information, most of which are already feasible in Scotland.

10 things that PCGs can do with good information

1 Targeted health promotion to localities.
2 Active management of chronic disease with automated quarterly reviews.
3 Real-time comparative clinical audits.
4 Comparison of doctor and nurse workloads.
5 Measurement of effectiveness of resource use by programme or practice.
6 Comparison of drugs costs with clinical outcomes at practice and PCG level.
7 Automated practice profiles.
8 Prediction of seasonal variation in demand by practice.
9 Research studies of impact of interventions on patient behaviour.
10 Impact of health promotion on deprived populations.

Exercise 16

Identify your own ten things that you would like to do, based upon my list. Identify the data required to achieve them in the table below.

Things to do	Data required

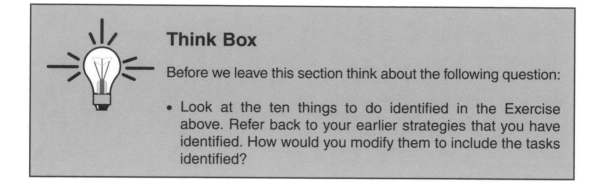

Think Box

Before we leave this section think about the following question:

- Look at the ten things to do identified in the Exercise above. Refer back to your earlier strategies that you have identified. How would you modify them to include the tasks identified?

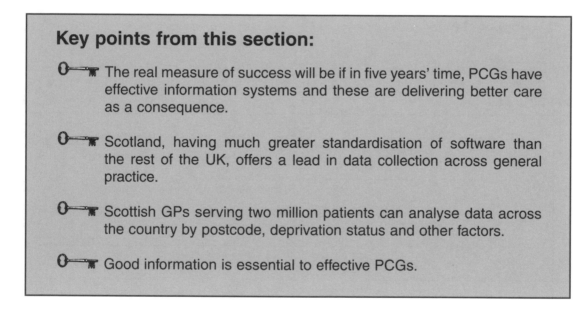

Key points from this section:

The real measure of success will be if in five years' time, PCGs have effective information systems and these are delivering better care as a consequence.

Scotland, having much greater standardisation of software than the rest of the UK, offers a lead in data collection across general practice.

Scottish GPs serving two million patients can analyse data across the country by postcode, deprivation status and other factors.

Good information is essential to effective PCGs.

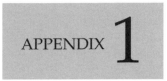

Where to find lots of

useful things for free

To accompany this book there is a Web site at www.lpsmh.freeserve.co.uk/Radcliffe

When I wrote the book, the following things could be found at the Web pages. Please bear in mind that the Web pages are dynamic and, therefore, they may have changed by the time you read this. Hopefully, they will have been added to rather than reduced in scope.

The Web site includes links to:

- *The New NHS* White Paper (1997)
- *Information for Health* (1998)
- Glossary of terms
- Rules for Accreditation for GP Systems version 4
- National data collection project: Collection of Health Data from General Practice (CHDGP)
- General Practice Information Maturity Model (GPIMM)
- Data Protection Registrar
- GPASS Data Evaluation Project
- The Department of Health Home Page
- Health Informatics Research Unit
- Public Access Medline
- *BMJ* on-line

In addition, the Web pages will contain updated information as things change.

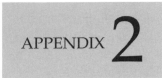

APPENDIX 2

Further reading for those
who can't swim

Non-swimmers who are therefore unable to surf the Net will find the key references below.

The New NHS White Paper (1997)

Department of Health (1997) *The New NHS*. HMSO, London.

The New NHS White Paper is the foundation document that lays out the roles and responsibilities of primary care groups.

Information for Health (1998)

Department of Health (1998) *Information for Health: The New NHS IM&T strategy*. HMSO, London.

This document is the IM&T strategy document that outlines future information strategy for the NHS. The strategy emphasises a shift away from technology to information itself and to clinical information from managerial information. However, to my way of thinking it is short on detail.

Glossary of terms

This glossary of terms is a very useful resource. It is provided as part of the Information for Health document listed above.

Rules for Accreditation for GP Systems

FHS (1997) *Rules for Accreditation for GP systems version 4*. Exeter. Contact FHS, an NHS agency, by telephone on 01392 206700 or at the address given in Appendix 3.

The rules for accreditation of GP systems contain lots of useful information, giving guidance as to what should be in a GP system.

National data collection project: Collection of Health Data from General Practice (CHDGP)

The CHDGP produces the following documents; if you do not have Web access write to the postal address given on p. 105.

CHDGP Guidelines

These are the 'rules' for the way in which the project is organised. Included are security and confidentiality safeguards, data recording guidelines, and an outline of analysis and feedback procedures. The Guidelines are organised as a series of fact-sheets. For a closer look, click on the Guidelines button under the map.

CHDGP Co-ordinator's Handbook

The Co-ordinator's Handbook was designed to help local scheme co-ordinators with the interpretation and practical use of the CHDGP Guidelines. It gives some interesting insights on facilitation, as well as on ways of managing data and information in general practice.

The Comparative Analysis Service Specification

Sets out the data to be extracted, security and confidentiality safeguards, and the analyses to be performed. You can get a copy by clicking on the button under the map.

The CHDGP project team may be contacted by telephone on 0115 919 4495 or at the address given in Appendix 3.

General Practice Information Maturity Model (GPIMM)

The following academic publications deal with the GPIMM:

1 Gillies AC (1998) Computers and the NHS: an analysis of their contribution to the past, present and future delivery of the National Health Service. *Journal of Information Technology.* **13** (8).
2 Gillies AC (1998) Towards a maturity model for computer usage in general practice. SIHCM '98, St Andrews, April.
3 Gillies AC (1998) Changes in information risks associated with the introduction of IT in primary care. Risk and Policy conference, Oxford, June.

The GPIMM model is copyright of the author. However, by buying the book, you have also bought a licence to use the GPIMM-CAPA tool. A copy of the CAPA tool is available on disk from the author for a handling charge of £15, for personal use only.

For general enquiries regarding GPIMM contact the author at the address given in Appendix 3.

The 1998 Data Protection Act

The following documents are available from the HMSO Bookstore in London (Tel: 0171-242 6393; full address in Appendix 3):

1 the 1998 Data Protection Act
2 data protection: the Government's proposals
3 EU data protection directive (95/46/EC)
4 the 1984 Data Protection Act.

GPASS Data Evaluation Project

Two publications illustrating results from the work on GPASS are:

Whitelaw FG, Taylor RJ, Nevin SL, Taylor MW, Milne RM, Watt AH (1996) Completeness and accuracy of morbidity and repeat prescribing records held on general practice computers in Scotland. *British Journal of General Practice*. **46**: 181–6.

Whitelaw FG, Nevin SL, Taylor RJ, Watt AH (1996) Morbidity and prescribing patterns for the middle-aged population of Scotland. *British Journal of General Practice*. **46**: 707–14.

For more up-to-date information, contact the project at the address given in Appendix 3.

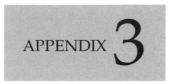

Useful addresses for non-swimmers

HMSO, for all government documents

London Stationery Office Bookshop
123 Kingsway
London WC2B 6PQ
Tel: 0171-242 6393
Fax: 0171-242 6394

CHDGP

CHDGP
Division of General Practice
University of Nottingham
Queen's Medical Centre
Nottingham NG7 2UH
Tel: 0115-919 4495
Fax: 0115-970 9389

Data Protection Registrar

The Office of the Data Protection Registrar
Wycliffe House
Water Lane
Wilmslow
Cheshire SK9 5AF
N.B. Documents available from the Stationery Office above

FHS, for rules for accreditation for GP systems

FHS
Hexagon House
Pynes Hill
Rydon Lane
Exeter
Devon EX2 5SE
Tel: 01392 206700
Fax: 01392 206946

GPASS Data Evaluation Project

GPASS Data Evaluation Project
Department of General Practice & Primary Care
University of Aberdeen
Foresterhill Health Centre
Westburn Road
Aberdeen AB25 2AY

GPIMM and the author

Professor Alan Gillies
Health Informatics Research Unit
Lancashire Postgraduate School of Medicine and Health
Harrington Building
University of Central Lancashire
Adelphi St
Preston PR1 2HE
Tel: 01772 893870
Fax: 01772 893871

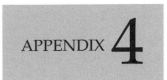

APPENDIX 4

The jargon buster

Algorithm

An algorithm is a series of steps, which we can use to achieve a process. It forms the basis for most structured computer programs. Algorithms are the subject of many weighty and incomprehensible tomes in computer science. However, the most common type of algorithm encountered in primary healthcare is a clinical guideline, which provides a series of steps to implement a clinical procedure.

Client server system

A client server system is a computer system organised in two parts. The client is a local computer which sends instructions for handling files, such as open, close, read, write, sort, to a remote server where the data is stored. A single client may access more than one server. For a full description see the 'File Server' entry in *Encyclopaedia of Computer Science* (3e). Chapman & Hall, London (1993).

Encryption

Encryption is the translation of messages into a form that is unintelligible to an outsider and is often used to improve security of information systems. The message is translated using an encryption algorithm to make it unintelligible. It can then only be decoded by use of the decryption algorithm, known as the key.

Electronic Health Record

The 1998 IM&T strategy describes the Electronic Health Record as a collection of all the various health data held about a patient by the NHS and other agencies, e.g. social services. It is an attractive proposition, but is some years away from realisation. It is best viewed as the Holy Grail towards which the NHS is working.

Elephant

Elephants are large grey animals found in Africa and Asia and in zoos in the rest of the world. The author alleges that many clinical computer systems resemble elephants in their ability to swallow huge amounts of data, lose most of it in their gizzards and excrete the rest as a useless pile of dung!

ICD9/10

ICD is the most common coding system used internationally for classifying disease for epidemiological purposes. Currently, the world is moving from ICD9 to ICD10. If Read is to be taken seriously beyond the NHS, then Read Codes must be able to be converted into ICD9 or 10 codes.

IM&T

Stands for information management and technology. Although it is commonly used in the NHS, it has to date been focused on IT rather than IM. Overseas academics tend to praise the NHS for its inclusion of IM issues. UK academics tend to ask 'Where?'. In fairness, the 1998 IM&T strategy starts to redress the balance.

Internet, The

The Internet is a global collection of computer networks to which anyone can gain access with a computer, a modem and a connection provided by an Internet service provider. The most common way in which people use the Internet is to access the World Wide Web, which is made up of billions of pages of information. The other common use is for electronic mail, allowing messages to be sent across the world.

Intranets

Intranets are networks within organisations designed to provide a kind of mini-Internet for that organisation. The NHSNet is an example of an organisation-wide Intranet.

Local Area Networks (LANs)

Local Area Networks (LANs) are small-scale networks, generally within one geographical location, providing access to an information system. For example, most GP patient systems operate as LANs to provide access to the system in a variety of locations throughout the surgery.

Millennium Bug, The

see Year 2000 compliance.

MIQUEST

The MIQUEST approach and Health Query Language is now used by projects in many areas of the UK NHS for collecting and analysing health data. It was originally developed between 1992 and 1994. The original MIQUEST project was jointly funded by the UK NHS Executive, Information Management Group and the former Northern RHA. It was established to facilitate the electronic collection of health data from commonly used general practice computer systems. To achieve this goal a structured Health Query Language (HQL) was defined. HQL is capable of expressing many current and potential requirements for data extraction from GP computer systems. For more information, visit the Clinical Information Consultancy Web Site at http://www.clinical-info.co.uk/miquest.htm#MiquestProject

NHSNet

NHSNet is the name of the NHS Intranet, i.e. a network to connect every site in the NHS. As you can imagine, this is a huge undertaking. It seems likely that every GP site will be physically connected during 1999, but it will be longer before meaningful information is flowing in large quantities.

Rules for Accreditation

These are the rules that all GP systems developers should follow, detailing the data to be collected, the way it should be accessed and the reports available. Currently in version 4, version 5 is under development and will be implemented later in 1999, with conformant systems expected in 2000. The scheme is administered by FHS, from whom more information is available.

Telemedicine

Telemedicine is literally the operation of medicine at a distance. It is a very trendy topic at present. In its simplest form, when a patient rings a surgery for a telephone consultation, this is telemedicine. However, current developments are much more ambitious, including consultations via video conferencing, transmission of test results including images via electronic links, and even experiments in remote surgery by use of robot arms controlled by a human surgeon at a distance. Scary. Currently, it is often a clever solution looking for a problem but developments in areas such as Queensland, Australia, where rural isolation is a real problem, are encouraging.

Wide Area Networks (WANs)

Wide Area Networks are large-scale networks, generally linking different geographical locations, providing access to an information system. WANs may be made up of linked LANs. For example a PCG might establish a WAN to link the GP systems in their area. The NHSNet is an example of an information system operating across a WAN. The Internet is arguably the biggest WAN in the world.

Year 2000 compliance
(also known as Y2K compliance)

The Year 2000 problem arises because in older systems, the year part of the date was often stored as two digits, rather than the full four. For example, 01/01/98 is assumed to be 1 January 1998. However, under this system, 01/01/00 is assumed to be 1 January 1900. This can cause computers to get confused, for example if a future appointment is set for 01/04/00 in 1999, it will be thought to be 99 years in the past not one year hence. Many functions such as those monitoring screening programs deduct one date from another. This may really confuse the computer, resulting in unpredictable behaviour. Year 2000 compliant systems have been checked to ensure that they can cope with the date change. To check that your system has been cleared as problem free, check the Information on RFA accreditation for your system, via the Web if possible. You can access this via the Web page associated with this book. All systems accredited to RFA4 have been certified as Year 2000 compliant, and should not be a problem.

For further information see: Gillies AC (1997) The year 2000 problem in general practice: an information management based analysis. *Journal of Health Informatics*. **3** (3&4): 147–53.

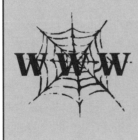 For a more complete glossary of terms see the glossary provided with the Information for Health document. This is available at: http://www.imt4nhs.exec.nhs.uk/strategy/full/glossary.htm, but I can't guarantee a jargon free zone!

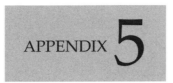

Model answers to
the exercises

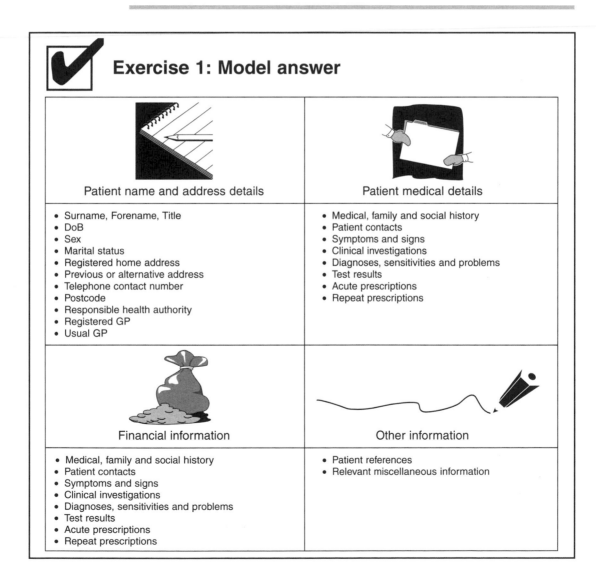

✔ Exercise 1: Model answer

Patient name and address details

- Surname, Forename, Title
- DoB
- Sex
- Marital status
- Registered home address
- Previous or alternative address
- Telephone contact number
- Postcode
- Responsible health authority
- Registered GP
- Usual GP

Patient medical details

- Medical, family and social history
- Patient contacts
- Symptoms and signs
- Clinical investigations
- Diagnoses, sensitivities and problems
- Test results
- Acute prescriptions
- Repeat prescriptions

Financial information

- Medical, family and social history
- Patient contacts
- Symptoms and signs
- Clinical investigations
- Diagnoses, sensitivities and problems
- Test results
- Acute prescriptions
- Repeat prescriptions

Other information

- Patient references
- Relevant miscellaneous information

Exercise 2: Model answer

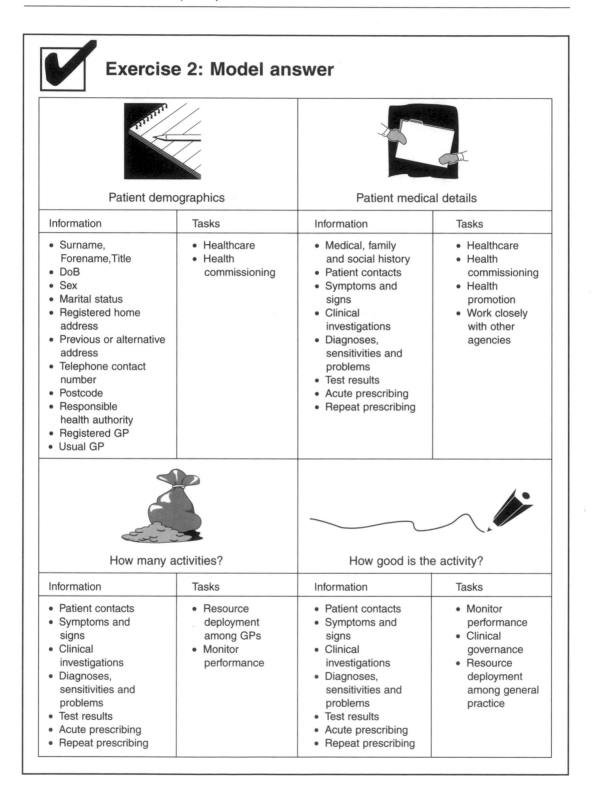

Patient demographics

Information	Tasks
• Surname, Forename, Title • DoB • Sex • Marital status • Registered home address • Previous or alternative address • Telephone contact number • Postcode • Responsible health authority • Registered GP • Usual GP	• Healthcare • Health commissioning

Patient medical details

Information	Tasks
• Medical, family and social history • Patient contacts • Symptoms and signs • Clinical investigations • Diagnoses, sensitivities and problems • Test results • Acute prescribing • Repeat prescribing	• Healthcare • Health commissioning • Health promotion • Work closely with other agencies

How many activities?

Information	Tasks
• Patient contacts • Symptoms and signs • Clinical investigations • Diagnoses, sensitivities and problems • Test results • Acute prescribing • Repeat prescribing	• Resource deployment among GPs • Monitor performance

How good is the activity?

Information	Tasks
• Patient contacts • Symptoms and signs • Clinical investigations • Diagnoses, sensitivities and problems • Test results • Acute prescribing • Repeat prescribing	• Monitor performance • Clinical governance • Resource deployment among general practice

✔ Exercise 3: Model answer

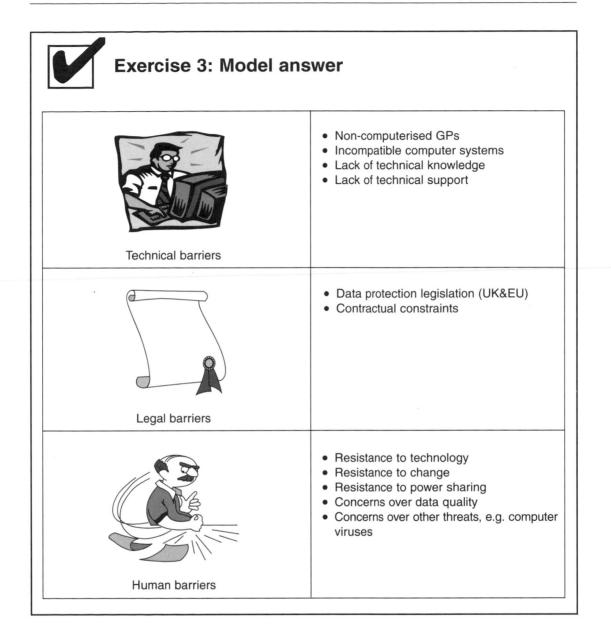

Technical barriers	• Non-computerised GPs • Incompatible computer systems • Lack of technical knowledge • Lack of technical support
Legal barriers	• Data protection legislation (UK&EU) • Contractual constraints
Human barriers	• Resistance to technology • Resistance to change • Resistance to power sharing • Concerns over data quality • Concerns over other threats, e.g. computer viruses

✔ Exercise 4: Model answer

Information in	Information out
• Name and number of practice	• Name and number of practice
• Address(es) of surgery	• Address(es) of surgery
• Telephone and fax numbers	• Telephone and fax numbers
• ~~Fund holding practice number*~~	• ~~Fund holding practice number*~~
• Name	• Name
• Professional ID numbers	• ~~Professional ID numbers~~
• Role details	• ~~Role details~~
• Contractual relationships with dates	• ~~Contractual relationships with dates~~
• Surname, Forename, Title	• Surname, Forename, Title
• DoB	• DoB
• Sex	• Sex
• Marital status	• Marital status
• New NHS number (10-digit)	• ~~New NHS number (10-digit)~~
• Old NHS number	• Old NHS number
• Registration type	• Registration type
• Registered home address	• Registered home address
• Previous or alternative address	• Previous or alternative address
• Telephone contact number	• Telephone contact number
• Postcode	• Postcode
• Responsible health authority	• Responsible health authority
• Registered GP	• Registered GP
• Usual GP	• Usual GP
• Dispensing status	• ~~Dispensing status~~
• ~~Rural practice information~~	• ~~Rural practice information~~
• Date of removal	• Date of removal
• Medical, family and social history	• Medical, family and social history
• Symptoms, signs and investigations	• Symptoms, signs and investigations
• Diagnoses, sensitivities and problems	• Diagnoses, sensitivities and problems
• All prescribable items	• All prescribable items
• Interactions and contraindications	• ~~Interactions and contraindications~~
• Doses and cautions	• Doses and cautions
• NHS price	• ~~NHS price~~
• NHS status and category	• NHS status and category

✔ Exercise 5: Model answer

Health authority systems	Links to GP systems
Items of service	✓
Patient registration details	✓
Pathology results	✓
PACT prescribing data	

✔ Exercise 6: Model answer

Strength/Weakness	Instance	Implication
✓ Storing information	Consultation	Updating patient record
✓ Sorting information	Consultation	Identifying patients
✓ Finding information	Consultation	Can find patient record
✓ Working quickly	Screening	Identify targets quickly
✓ Doing what they are told	Protocols	Follow rules accurately
✓ Talking to other computers	Communications	Seamless EHR
✓ Passing on information to other computers quickly	Communications	Transfer of images, etc.
✓ Adding up and doing other sums	Research/Audit	Analysis of data
✓ Producing pretty graphs from numbers	Research/Audit	Presentation of data
✓ Sitting there and not getting impatient whilst waiting for the next instruction	Consultation	Unobtrusive
✗ Not being intelligent	Data entry	Won't correct user errors
✗ Computers do what you say, not what you want	Data entry	Won't correct user errors
✗ They don't use judgement	Guideline/ Protocols	Inflexible
✗ Bad at communicating with people	General usage	Unpopularity with users
✗ Applying contextual information	Consultation	Output needs human filter
✗ Working with fuzzy data, e.g. diagnoses	Coding	Can lead to spurious precision
✗ Remembering when power is switched off	General usage	Need for backups
✗ Working the way people work	General usage	Unpopularity with users
✗ Telling when people are lying	Consultation	Output needs human filter
✗ Using common sense, they don't have any!	Consultation	Output needs human filter

✔ Exercise 7: Model answer

1 How about
TM3	Injury due to legal intervention by blunt object
UA123	Accidental poisoning/exposure to sedative/hypnotic in a sport/ athletic area
TM81	Legal execution by beheading
XA2NT	Eating own flesh.

2 I love Read Codes because they make Department of Health circulars seem interesting by comparison.

✔ Exercise 8: Model answer

Clinical areas covered	Clinical terms identified	Read Codes
Diabetes: morbidity	Diabetes mellitus	C10+
Diabetes: monitoring	Diabetes monitored	66A.
Diabetes: treatment	Diet	66A3.
	Oral	66A4.
	Insulin	66A5.
Diabetes: management	Shared care	66S9.
	GP care	66S2.
	Specialist (i.e. hospital) care	
Diabetes: indicators	HbA1c levels	42W+
	Serum fructosamine	44Z1+
	Urine protein levels	467+
Diabetes: complications	Diabetes & eye manifestation	C105+
	Nephropathy	C104+
	Neuropathy	C106+
	Peripheral circulatory disease	C107+
	Hypoglycaemia	C112